The
Learning
Disability
Myth

The Learning Disability Myth

Understanding and overcoming your child's diagnosis of Dyspraxia, Dyslexia, Tourette's syndrome of childhood, ADD, ADHD and OCD

DR **ROBIN PAUC**

WITH JACQUELINE BURNS

BP53

To our children's futures

First published in the USA in 2006 by
Virgin Books Ltd
Thames Wharf Studios
Rainville Road
London W6 9HA

Distributed in the USA by
Holtzbrinck Publishers, LLC
175 Fifth Avenue
New York
NY 10010
USA
www.holtzbrinckus.com

Library of Congress Cataloging-in-Publication Data

ISBN 0 7535 1127 4
ISBN 9 780753 511275

Typeset by Phoenix Photosetting, Chatham, Kent
Printed and bound in the USA

10/15/07

CONTENTS

FOREWORD

by Professor Frederick Robert Carrick,
The Carrick Institute, Cape Canaveral

When asked to write a foreword to Dr. Robin Pauc's book, I was concerned that this might be just another of the mass of similar works about learning and behavioral disorders in childhood. Instead, I was pleased to realize that his work is one that is uniquely addressed to parents and educators who are directly and personally challenged by a variety of syndromes affecting children.

Dr. Pauc's essential book presents us with questions that are very personal and to the point, including "Is that *my* child?" Not only does Dr. Pauc direct us to ask the question, he gives us direction and guidance when we are faced with the uncomfortable conclusion, "Yes, that *is* my child." As a neurologist, when reading this book I additionally felt myself presented with a concept that all children are "mine" and that the medical and sociological consequences of the disorders discussed by Dr. Pauc are very personal.

While Pauc's contribution describes the syndromes of dyspraxia, dyslexia, ADD, ADHD, OCD and Tourette's syndrome of childhood similarly to other works, he presents a novel hypothesis for their cause, and treatment for the disorders. He details the types of examinations that parents must demand of their doctors for their children and then identifies a variety of treatments which are easily incorporated into a family-based treatment model. This work therefore empowers the parent and makes him or her part of both the diagnosis and the therapy.

This book presents the common groupings of learning and behavioral disorders of childhood in their reality as symptoms rather than as diseases. He also discusses the things that can go wrong within a child's environment or nutrition and gives direction in how to direct change. He gives realistic hope to the parent, supported by his personal success in the treatment of numerous children who suffer with these syndromes.

In this book Dr. Pauc presents a model of development that he has called *bpoptosis*. While the intricate program of cell death and proliferation of apoptosis describes both the intentional and unintentional death of cells in development, Pauc's bpoptosis is central to the life of cells. His theory embraces concepts that are interesting, plausible, but most importantly applicable in the diagnosis and treatment of childhood brain-based problems. His work echoes the concept of life and development, rather than disease and death.

This book is written for the parents and teachers who must deal with the personal reality of the increasing numbers of learning and behavioral disorders in children. It is well written and presents a reasonable science in terms that are understandable for those without a neuroscience background. Dr. Pauc allows the reader to realize that they suffer with their child and that the parent must play an integral role in both the diagnosis and treatment of learning disorders.

Professor Frederick Robert Carrick
Professor Emeritus of Neurology
The Carrick Institute
Cape Canaveral
USA

INTRODUCTION

WHY THIS BOOK IS DIFFERENT

The Learning Disability Myth is, in a particular way, different from most books published on learning disabilities and contains very positive information for parents and carers of children with learning disabilities.

We are living in a time in which perceptions about learning and behavioral difficulties are beginning to change. Even so, you may be wondering why we need yet another book on the problems surrounding learning disabilities, considering the proliferation of books on the subject.

It is my belief, however, that you do need this book, because *The Learning Disability Myth* is a groundbreaking work, with a revolutionary new treatment. And I hope that once you've read what is within these pages you will be convinced too.

I have been a functional neurologist for eight years and my work involves looking at the living brain to understand how it functions. The breakthrough in my work came at my clinic, Tinsley House, when I made a link between what happens when there is a problem in the development of brain cells that happens in all children at about four months of age and the effect that has on a child's developing brain.

I then realized that, by stimulating the area of the brain that is affected, we should see an improvement in a child's ability to do the tasks they have previously found difficult. The results were very exciting, even more so than I had hoped.

The good news for parents, therefore, is that something can be done about their children's learning and behavioral difficulties and that there are practical steps you can take to lessen the likelihood of your child suffering from these symptoms. By combining a program of brain-stimulating exercises and putting the child on a healthier diet—I have included a 14-day menu and some sample recipes to guide parents—I have achieved what I believe to be a near-total solution with every child.

In a nutshell this book will:

- explain the new discovery that all human babies are born "prematurely" in the sense that they are "incomplete" at birth with a further crucial stage of development taking place at four months of age;
- reveal how a problem with the second-wave of nerve cell generation is the cause of a child's developmental delay; this is cutting-edge neurology and probably the single greatest breakthrough in pediatric neurology this decade; it is so unique that I have created a new word to describe it: *bpoptosis* (I have also included a glossary at the back to explain some of the terms);
- show how the symptoms of developmental delay are related to specific areas of the brain;
- carefully detail how the child should be examined correctly to get to the heart of the problem;
- provide a treatment plan that works, including an eating plan and some exercises;
- detail the wider implications in this work.

If left untreated, I have discovered that these learning disabilities will have a much more significant impact on the functioning of our society than might be superficially apparent. Unresolved, these children who have learning disabilities will go into adulthood still suffering from the problem itself—which is bad enough—but also from the complications that cause them. I finish the book by explaining what the ramifications are and how we might tackle this issue.

As you may have noticed, the term "delay" implies that the problem is one of being stalled or behind, rather than being a permanent problem. That is absolutely correct. This book offers you a *treatment* for learning disabilities. And that is why this book may be one of the most important ones on the subject that you will retain on your shelves.

Finally, as already indicated, the treatment for developmental delay syndrome, which is the subject of this book, was pioneered at the Tinsley House Clinic in the UK. We are now planning to set up clinics in the United States and internationally, and you will be able to find the latest news about this at my website (www.tinsleyhouseclinic.com).

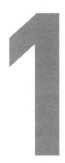

LEARNING DISABILITIES: THE BACKGROUND

In this chapter we will cover:

- the background to learning disabilities;
- what to expect of your child;
- what to expect of this book.

THE BACKGROUND

Learning and behavioral difficulties have had an adverse effect on the lives of millions of children around the world.

In the UK, nearly one in five children experiences some sort of learning disability or behavioral problem. Based on the 2001 government census I estimate that there are potentially more than two and a quarter million children in the UK with problems. These children experience significant problems at home and at school every day. This is of huge concern for their parents and a key issue for teachers whose classrooms are more often than not suffering from overcrowding.

Worst of all, the children affected are not living their lives as happily as they could be. Daily life is tough for them.

The dark past of learning and behavioral difficulties

In the distant past if a child did not do well at school they were often viewed in a very poor light and described in negative terms. They were thought to be slow, lazy, sometimes labeled as "not right in the head" or all of these things. The other unenlightened yet accepted views included putting the blame on poor parenting. None of these "diagnoses" helped the child.

Parents were alone in dealing with their children's problem and perhaps marginalized and pitied for having an "idiot" child. As a parent it would have been difficult not to blame yourself and to be blamed by others. At Tinsley House Clinic the mothers I see may particularly be suffering varying degrees of guilt. They often blame themselves, wondering if it was something that they did wrong in pregnancy. However, in the vast majority of cases, those mothers could not have done anything more to care for their unborn child.

Fortunately those dark days of ignorance about learning disabilities are over. Instead, over the last twenty or thirty years we have seen a shift toward greater understanding and increased sympathy for children who find reading, learning and daily life so difficult. Clearly this is a change for the better.

Not only have attitudes changed for the better, but the government has also stepped in, and now you can expect help from the medical and educational systems. This is a great relief for parents and a vast improvement for the children concerned.

The main shift began when the medical establishment made attempts to diagnose and label learning disabilities and behavioral problems. Their intention was to solve the child's problem. It was thought that from this starting point—figuring out what was wrong and giving it a name—the beginnings of a treatment for these problems would emerge.

The labels used are: attention deficit hyperactivity disorder (ADHD), attention deficit disorder (ADD), dyslexia, dyspraxia, obsessive-compulsive disorder (OCD), autism and Tourette's syndrome.

These labels are universally used and many people find them useful. There are a number of reasons for this. The key reason is that the help and support given to a child depends upon the child's being diagnosed and labeled by the education and medical systems.

It also helps parents. To have a name for what is wrong gives them a sense that they know what the problem is and that there is a treatment for that particular condition. They feel less helpless and alone. For the child, they're probably simply grateful for the extra help and attention they receive instead of being pushed harder.

To insure that a child receives good support from the school and so that something is done about the child's problem, the condition needs to be officially recognized. Many parents are upset to hear that their child is dyslexic but are relieved to have the problem defined. If the problem has a name—the reasoning goes—then someone has to, and will, do something about it.

Each condition will be fully explained in Chapter 2, but for now I'd like to ask you to consider your child and what their developmental experience might be.

WHAT TO EXPECT OF YOUR CHILD

All children are different and develop at different rates, so you may well ask, "How do I know if anything is wrong?" Are they perhaps just a little late developing, or is there a problem that needs attention?

You may have noticed problems with your child already, or perhaps you are just worried that they're not keeping up with their peers. Perhaps they were slow to walk, or talk, or they behave in a way that is different from other children. Whatever you are concerned about, this section is to help you to think about and detect signs of problems as early on as possible.

At Tinsley House Clinic we believe in addressing problems as quickly as possible. The sooner your child's problem is detected, the sooner it can be fixed. If possible it is better to have a child properly diagnosed and treated before they start school. If nothing is done until they start to fall behind, then struggling with a learning disability and also having to catch up can leave them, in terms of learning achievement, behind their peers. This could mean that they will suffer from low self-esteem and the unnecessary stigma of being at the bottom of the class. If your child has already started school, don't worry—it is not too late to make changes and this book can help you do that.

I am not going to give you a full description of the stages of child development here, but rather a quick checklist so that you can see if there may be problems with your child. I will briefly explain what you should expect of a child who is developing at an average rate.

Developmental milestones

Each child enters the world with a set of primitive reflexes designed specifically to help them survive. For instance, if you stroke a baby's cheek they will turn their head toward you, hoping to find a nipple. You may not be aware of these reflexes but your doctor will check to see if they have disappeared, as they should do, between six and twelve months.

Here is a brief checklist of some developmental milestones that are often found at certain stages of infancy.

- *Important note: all children will differ in their development, some will be faster, some slower, so this should simply be regarded as a guide for the "average" child, and nothing more. There is no need to worry if you find that for any reason your child's behavior does not conform to any of these milestones. This is not intended to be a set of hard and fast rules, but merely broad indications of what you might expect to find.*

By six weeks the child may be able to lift their head and produce a proper smile (not that strange look usually due to gas).

By four months the child may be attempting to grasp large objects, laugh and show obvious pleasure in response to familiar toys or people.

By five months the child may be playing with their toes, using both hands to manipulate objects and be making those funny little noises we all love—"Ah, goo" etc.

By six months the child may be able to sit unaided, roll over, be making even more noises and, unfortunately, be able to let you know just what they don't like.

By eight months the child may be combining syllables—"dada," "mama"—and may be starting to understand the meaning of "No."

By ten months the child may be crawling, be able to stand while holding on to something, to use thumb and finger to pick up small objects (developing manual dexterity), and to wave goodbye to people.

By one year the child may be walking and have a collection of single words that people other than family members understand. By this stage they may be starting to understand what the names of objects mean.

By fifteen months the child may have more words, be able to imitate others, and point to objects that they want.

By two years the child may be putting two words together and be able to follow simple commands. Unfortunately, they may also have now mastered the stairs.

By two and a half years the child may be potty-trained by day (with occasional bed-wetting incidents).

By three years the child may be making simple sentences and may no longer wet the bed at night.

See the References/Further reading section at the back of this book for further information and guidance on child development.

The following questionnaire is taken from one used at Tinsley House Clinic for children of four years and upwards, and I include it here to help you consider possible factors you may need to be aware of about your child. These answers may provide clues as to what is wrong with your child but it should only be used as a rough guide and is not a replacement for a proper diagnosis. Simply answer the questions, add up the points and read the result below.

IS THAT MY CHILD?—QUESTIONNAIRE

1 **Is there a family history of any learning or behavioral problems?**
   Yes = 10 points, No = 0 points
2 **Were you and the baby fit and well during the pregnancy?**
   Yes = 0 points, No = 1 point
3 **Did the pregnancy go to full term?**
   Yes = 0 points, No = 2 points

4   Was the delivery natural or assisted (ventouse, Caesarean or forceps)?
Natural = 0 points, Assisted = 5 points

5   Was there any concern over fetal distress?
Yes = 5 points, No = 0 points

6   When did your child sit unaided?
Six months or earlier = 0, Later than six months = 2 points

7   Did your child crawl?
Yes = 0 points, No = 2 points

8   When did your child walk?
One year or earlier = 0 points, Later than one year = 1 point

9   In the first year did your child have a collection of single words?
Yes = 0 points, No = 1 point

10 In the second year did your child put two words together?
Yes = 0 points, No = 1 point

11 By the third year was your child making mini-sentences?
Yes = 0 points, No = 1 point

12 When was your child potty-trained by day?
Two and a half years or earlier = 0 points, Later than two and a half years = 1 point

13 When was your child no longer wetting the bed at night?
Three years or earlier = 0 points, Later than three years = 2 points

14 Have there been any bed-wetting incidents since?
Yes = 1 point, No = 0 points

15 Has your child ever soiled?
Yes = 2 points, No = 0 points

16 Does your child have problems with reading/writing?
Yes = 2 points, No = 0 points

17 Does your child have problems in concentrating?
Yes = 1 point, No = 0 points

18 Is your child ever hyperactive?
Yes = 2 points, No = 0 points

19 How is your child's short-term memory?
Good = 0 points, Poor = 1 point

20 Has your child ever had any rituals or obsessions?
Yes = 3 points, No = 0 points

21 Has your child ever had any involuntary movements, tics, excessive blinking, grimacing, or made repeated sounds?
Yes = 5 points, No = 0 points

22 Is your child, or was your child ever, clumsy or accident-prone?
Yes = 2 points, No = 0 points

Results

15 points or less means that you have very little to worry about
16–29 points means that there is a high probability of developmental delay
30 points or more means that a developmental delay is virtually certain

WHAT TO EXPECT OF THIS BOOK

As I mentioned in the Introduction, the problems in development of new brain cells four months after birth—which I discuss in more detail in Chapter 4—is the cause of learning and behavioral difficulties, which should be more correctly termed Developmental Delay Syndrome (DDS). Irrespective of how high the score in the questionnaire above might be, however, the good news for parents and all concerned is that something can be done to help eradicate learning and behavioral difficulties, and *The Learning Disability Myth* offers practical help. By combining a program of stimulating the brain through both mental and physical exercises, and putting the child on a healthier diet, I have seen remarkable improvements in every child I've treated. Most often, their symptoms have disappeared entirely. The same can be done for your child.

The problem that the majority of children have is of being stalled and delayed in their development, rather than being subject to a permanent disorder, which is why I have reclassified learning disabilities and behavioral problems as developmental delay syndromes. I'll explain more about this in Chapter 3.

Chapter 2 will describe in detail the differently named learning disabilities. If you already know what your child's problem is then you can go straight to that condition. If you are unsure, you may have to read through the section on each condition to identify characteristics that may apply to your child. The key here is that whatever you know about your child's problem, it is best to keep an open mind until a complete diagnosis has been made (for more about this, see Chapters 7 and 8).

The following chapter will help you to start to ask yourself, "*Is that my child?*" and to begin the process of finding a solution for them.

2

THE CONDITIONS AND LABELS DEFINED AND EXPLAINED

Currently, when children are diagnosed with a learning disability they are pigeonholed based on the most obvious symptom and the condition that they might fit into.

This chapter will explain each of the conditions as they are commonly known, and give their definitions. I have stuck to the known names for each problem, but I want to mention at this point that I use the term developmental delay syndrome to describe all of these learning and behavioral difficulties (the reasons for this will be explained in Chapter 3).

This chapter will also include information about the day-to-day difficulties experienced by the children affected and how the medical and educational systems support them and work with them.

As I will discuss more fully in Chapter 3, because all learning disabilities are caused by a problem in the development of certain brain cells, all children with a learning disability will experience more than one condition. This may sound alarming—and will be explained fully below—but the more we understand that this is the case, the easier it is to treat *all* the conditions. So, when reading through the symptoms of each problem, it might help you to keep an open mind and think, "Is that my child?"

Also in this chapter—and throughout the book—you'll find a series of case histories of children treated at Tinsley House Clinic (the names of the children have been changed to protect their identity). Each case is presented under a heading that reflects the presenting diagnosis provided by either a health professional or the parent. In each case you will see that the predominant disorder does not appear alone and that fully understanding what is wrong with your child is more complicated than saying your child is dyslexic or has ADHD.

Now let's look at the learning and behavioral difficulties we will be discussing in this book.

DYSLEXIA

Dyslexia is defined as the impaired ability to read, spell and write words, despite the ability to see and recognize letters. It can include the following:

Delayed speech

The generally accepted rule of thumb of "normal" development is to expect a child to use single words in the first year, two words together during the second year and mini-sentences in the third year. Any delays here should be noticed by your doctor or by the health visitor during developmental checks. If your child has a problem here they may be referred—at about four years old or above—to a speech therapist.

Stuttering

Early onset stuttering—that is more or less from when your child first starts to construct sentences—is not uncommon. The act of constructing a sentence takes place in the left side of the brain. The gaps between words and the lilt of language—prosody—is a right-brain activity. Ninety-eight percent of children with learning disabilities have problems predominantly in the right side of the brain and it is probably a delay in maturation here that causes this problem.

Recurrent ear infections

Middle ear infections, eczema and asthma are so common in association with learning and behavioral problems that they could be classed as a symptom. Again this points to a problem on the right side of the brain, as part of the control system for the immune system lives there (though it seems mainly to affect the ears).

Poor coordination

Although this is often included in the broad definition of dyslexia, poor coordination is in reality labeled dyspraxia, which I discuss later. Not only is dyspraxia included with dyslexia, but also dyspraxia is further subdivided into the various forms it may take:

- dressing dyspraxia, e.g. tying shoelaces
- feeding dyspraxia, i.e. a messy eater
- poor handwriting associated with cramp in the hand and arm due to excessive gripping of the pencil

Humans—and the great apes to a lesser extent—have a specialized area of the brain that has evolved in parallel with an increasing skill with their hands to allow delicate finger control for such activities as writing or painting. If this specialized area of the brain is not working as it should, another area on the opposite side of the hemisphere of the brain takes over which unfortunately can only produce a power grip and hence too much force. This is why some children cannot hold a pen properly and cannot write very well, if at all.

Confusion over left- and right-handedness

In theory the left side of the brain should mature first, and this is thought to be why most people are right-handed (the left part of the brain controls the right side of the body in this case). There is a wave of special brain cells that develops in humans four months after birth (explained fully in Chapter 4). They are present on both sides of the brain but are concentrated on the right side, so can spur on left-handedness if there has been any delay in development of the brain up to this point. This can easily lead to confusion and the child ends up not sure which is left and which is right, and/or which hand to use.

Difficulty reading and/or the letters appear to move on the page

In a recent study, 58 percent of the children attending my clinic were found to have accommodation/convergence failure. That is, if you have to look at something close-up as when reading, your eyes have to move inwards toward your nose so that you can focus on the word you are reading. In the majority of cases of children with learning or behavioral difficulties, the left eye fails to do this, and as all the children in this particular study denied having double vision, then the information from the left eye must be ignored by the brain. This not only causes problems for the brain in terms of processing the information which should be coming from both eyes, but also makes tracking across the page very difficult, often leading to what is called nystagmus. This flickering of the eye to and fro is interpreted by the brain not as your eye moving from side to side, but that what you are looking at is moving. This is the same illusion of movement that happens after drinking too much alcohol.

Interestingly, very few opticians test for the convergence failure, described above, which is something of a concern when so many children have this problem. Apart from this, a significant number of children have poor vision on testing, which rapidly improves once the brain's developmental delay is addressed.

YOU CAN TEST FOR CONVERGENCE YOURSELF

Take a pencil in your right hand and hold it up vertically, level with your child's eyes and roughly 18 inches in front of them. Now move it slowly toward your child's nose, telling them to look at it all the time. The eyes should start to move in at the same time and should be able to continue looking at the pencil even when it is only a few inches away from the nose. A delay in either eye starting to move in or an eye that moves out to the side while the pencil is still close to the nose is a sign of accommodation/convergence failure.

Light sensitivity

A small percentage of children diagnosed with dyslexia are hypersensitive to light, where just a quick flash of light into the eyes during the examination is enough to cause the eyes to stream. Children with this problem often complain about bright sunlight or the headlights of approaching cars at night. This is generally a brain stem problem that runs in tandem with delayed development of the brain. Although this may sound quite alarming, it is not a cause for concern in this context as it will improve in parallel with the improvement of the developmental delay.

Coexisting conditions

I have described how various forms of dyspraxia are often lumped in with dyslexia; however, research has shown that 40 percent of children with dyslexia also have attention deficit disorder (ADD) and/or attention deficit hyperactive disorder (ADHD). We will see shortly that ADD and ADHD are also closely associated with other forms of behavioral problems.

Dyslexia: the story so far

Government figures estimate that in the total population, 5–20 percent of the population has a language-based learning disability. Of those 70–80 percent have deficits in reading, with dyslexia being the most common cause for reading problems.

Because of the sheer numbers of people affected, dyslexia attracts a lot of media attention. In the UK a television program on dyslexia in 2005 resulted in 275,000 people calling ITV to get further information and help. Clearly there are a lot of people out there who need help; help that they are not currently receiving even with extra school assistance and existing treatments.

The term dyslexia was first used over a hundred years ago in 1887 by Rudolph Berlin (the word comes from the Greek *dys* meaning difficult and *lesicos/lexicos* pertaining to words). The puzzle that led to dyslexia being identified was why many otherwise intelligent children could not read or else could only read very poorly. However, as any parent with a child with dyslexia will know, trying to find out what dyslexia is exactly can prove to be an insurmountable problem. There are endless books on the subject but none that provides an accurate description or diagnosis, and certainly none which provides any hope of a solution.

Despite this confusion there is some comfort in the label, mainly because, when children are evaluated for special education needs by the education system, they receive extra help at school. This reassures parents because they feel they do not have to shoulder the burden alone, and it helps teachers who find it difficult to give one child (or perhaps more) extra attention when they have a full classroom.

SPECIAL EDUCATION

Both state and federal laws exist for the benefit of children with learning disabilities. While assessment methods may vary from state to state, by law in the United States all special needs children must be accomodated in the public schools. If you feel your child may have special educational needs, speak to your child's teacher or ask to meet with the special education coordinator of your local school district.

I believe that the labels can be misleading and that we should use the general term Developmental Delay. However, many teachers and parents understandably fear that if we take away these labels then we also take away children's hard-won entitlement to help and support in the classroom. In a UK TV documentary, *Dispatches,* aired in September 2005 one parent—describing the relief parents feel when they have an official diagnosis of dyslexia— said, "Once it's in black-and-white you can't ignore it." So in many ways it is not surprising that parents and teachers were alarmed at the suggestion in that same program, by Professor Julian Elliott of Durham University, UK, that the label dyslexia is a myth and that it doesn't exist—or, more accurately, that the term is not useful.

After making a presentation to a teacher's conference, Professor Elliott was criticized by teachers who were incensed that what he had said would mean that the support for which the children's parents had fought so hard would be removed. The parents, in turn, were also devastated.

My opinion is that, although I am in agreement with Professor Elliott that these conditions do not exist as separate conditions, these children do still have a need that should be addressed and they should receive back-up in the form of special education classes.

DYSPRAXIA

To make matters more complicated, we now have a relatively new term—dyspraxia—which is often applied to children with developmental/learning disabilities, and is sometimes quite wrongly interchanged with dyslexia as if it were the same thing.

Dyspraxia is defined as a partial loss of the ability to perform coordinated acts. At one time called "clumsy child syndrome," it is an inability or difficulty in planning and carrying out planned movements or in orientating yourself within your environment. For a child this means that daily tasks like tying shoelaces and feeding themselves, and fun things like riding a bike, are enormous challenges. Not knowing exactly where you are in space means that you constantly bump into things or drop things.

In the context of learning and behavioral disabilities, the term developmental dyspraxia should be used to cover the signs and symptoms that occur in these young children. The condition includes:

- poor balance
- difficulties in both fine (such as writing and painting) and gross (such as running and jumping) motor skills
- problems with vision
- problems with motor planning and perception, i.e. preparing a movement and awareness of where you are in space
- poor bodily awareness
- difficulty with reading, writing and speech
- poor social skills
- emotional/behavioral problems

Already we can see an intriguing overlap between developmental dyspraxia and dyslexia as described above. In a recent study completed at Tinsley House Clinic it was found that every child included in the study had varying degrees of developmental dyspraxia, regardless of the initial primary diagnosis—dyslexia, ADD, ADHD, OCD or Tourette's syndrome of childhood.

It is the right side of the brain that deals with your position in space and it is this side of the brain that shows developmental delay in nearly all (98 percent) of children with problems. The brain changes the side of dominant activity roughly every 90 minutes and that is why when traveling a familiar route you either can't remember driving through a particular village or you notice an old cottage that you don't remember seeing before. When the right brain is dominant you only see the big picture—you are on autopilot—but

The Human Brain Viewed from Above

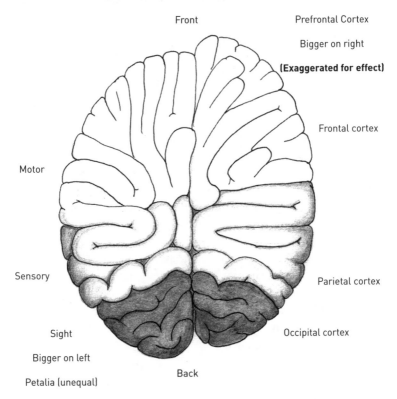

Front

Prefrontal Cortex

Bigger on right

(Exaggerated for effect)

Frontal cortex

Motor

Sensory

Parietal cortex

Sight

Occipital cortex

Bigger on left

Petalia (unequal)

Back

when the left brain takes over you notice every detail in your immediate environment.

Aspects of the functional dominance (one side dominating the other) of the cerebral hemispheres are evident in children with developmental delays and manifest themselves as a reluctance to meet change. With all of us, when we enter a new situation, the right side of the brain assesses the situation as to whether it is safe or not; it is the approach and/or withdrawal center checking first and foremost that we are safe.

We are all familiar with this, for instance when we enter a new dentist's waiting room. Firstly, we take a quick look around the room and then take a seat. Only after a few moments do we start looking around the room noticing the details, as our left brain takes over once our right brain has decided we are safe. A child with a developmental delay has a right brain that is under-functioning and so every situation is a challenge both in terms of fitting into the new environment and in assessing its potential dangers.

Dyspraxia—Dan, aged seven

*Dan, having been diagnosed with dyspraxia, was brought to see me by his mother. There was no history of dyspraxia, dyslexia or any other learning disability in the family. The pregnancy went to full-term but some help was needed with the delivery. No fetal distress was reported and Dan reached his developmental milestones at the right time with the exception of **bladder control**, which was a little late.*

*No problems were evident until Dan had to do things for himself, when it became clear that he had a **dressing dyspraxia**. That is, left to his own devices Dan could not work out what to put where and in which order. He had always been a little clumsy but increasingly this became a major problem in his life. It seemed as though he had a real problem fitting himself into his environment.*

*He had always been a **poor sleeper**, with difficulties getting off to sleep and being aroused from it by any sounds in the house.*

*Once at school, more problems became apparent as he took everything literally, could not place a drawing, or indeed writing, within the confines of the page and was well behind his peers in both **reading and writing**.*

*On further questioning it became clear that Dan still had some problems with **bladder control**, particularly when tired; he also had some minor **obsessional traits**, a poor **short-term memory** and serious **problems concentrating** on the matter in hand.*

On examination it was clear that the dyspraxia was the most prominent sign, but aspects of dyslexia, ADD and some obsessional traits were also evident. Bed-wetting is a very good indicator of reduced brain function associated with delayed maturation and the other signs and symptoms strongly indicated a right hemisphericity, that is, an immaturity or delayed development of the right hemisphere of the brain. What I found when I examined him confirmed my initial diagnosis based on the questions I had asked about his and his family's history during the consultation. The brain will be covered in more depth in Chapter 4, but briefly in this case the left cerebellum was grossly under-functioning which, together with areas of the right cerebral cortex, were generating the mixture of signs and symptoms which I have termed a developmental delay syndrome (see Chapter 3).

Following a session of treatment at the clinic using physical therapy to send messages to the left cerebellum, he was sent home with a simple yet highly challenging exercise for the developmental delay to be performed twice a day for the next two weeks. This consisted of no more than walking up and down three steps of the stairs with his hands by his side, eyes closed and head in the neutral position, i.e. in the normal position looking straight ahead. (If you think that is easy, try it, but make sure you have a responsible adult on hand to catch you should you fall, as many children do.)

At the following visit his mother reported that Dan's dyspraxia had dramatically improved, his strength had increased and he was managing to do things he had struggled with before. After his fourth treatment every single aspect of his problem was showing marked improvement. Both Dan and his mother were delighted.

CHECKING AND MONITORING FOR IMPROVEMENTS AT TINSLEY HOUSE CLINIC

An important part of the treatment we provide is monitoring progress. We need to document all signs of improvement and gather this information from various sources. Usually the parents are the first to comment on the little things they have noticed, but this is quickly followed by reports from other significant people in the child's life including relatives, friends of the family and schoolteachers.

The subjective findings are provided by constant reassessment, with the child not only being retested at each visit but also between individual treatments. This constant monitoring not only allows the practitioner to see how the child is progressing, but is a great encouragement to the parents.

The best measure of all has to be when children tell me how well they are coping, how well they are doing at school and how different they are feeling. Little else really matters.

Verbal dyspraxia—Marcus, aged four and a half

*Marcus was brought to see me by his mother because of slow **speech development**, which had further deteriorated following a bout of ear* infections so that he no longer spoke at all. At the time of consultation Marcus was four and a half but appeared much younger due to a slowed physical development.

On questioning it was revealed that Marcus **wet the bed** every night, had frequent accidents by day, **shunned affection** and was basically **a loner**, avoiding contact with other children.

On examination he was unable to stand upright with his eyes closed, had reduced reflexes, an inability to converge his eyes for close vision, and was exceedingly dyspraxic. The first treatment at the clinic simply involved—much to his and his mother's surprise—pulling his left toes and fingers, which sends a barrage of messages to the cerebellum and shocks the system. He was sent home with a simple exercise to practice three times a day and a list of foods, additives and sweeteners to avoid (see Chapters 9–11).

The changes in Marcus were spectacular to say the least. Following his second treatment at the clinic Marcus climbed into bed with his mother and cuddled her. His mother cried, having never experienced any expression of affection from him before. On his third visit to the clinic he started talking, albeit quietly at first, and his mother reported that he was now potty-trained by day. During the next two weeks he no longer wet the beds at night and was constantly asking his mother if he could go next door to play with the neighbor's children.

I monitored Marcus over a period of months, mainly by e-mail reports from his mother, and have been delighted by his continued progress and the speed at which he has made up lost ground. To his mother's immense relief, Marcus will be absolutely fine.

Teenagers can be helped too—Lenny, aged fifteen

Lenny, a very pleasant boy aged fifteen, came to see me having already been diagnosed with dyslexia. Twenty minutes later, following a simple yet highly accurate computer-generated test, no dyslexic traits were detected.

On talking at length with his mother it became clear that on her husband's side of the family there were many male members with distinct learning disabilities. The pregnancy had gone well, the labor had been short and the delivery uncomplicated until it was realized that the cord was around the baby's neck, causing **fetal distress**.

Lenny's progress was unremarkable, perhaps a little delayed, and *no real problems were encountered until he started school. In the formal learning situation he failed, unable to learn anything except by constant repetition. He excelled at sports and was popular among his peers but privately was deeply unhappy, with little or no self-esteem.*

Testing showed that the left cerebellum was under-functioning and the right cerebral hemisphere was well below the left in terms of processing speed, suggesting developmental delay. Lenny was treated with the help of a computer program that he could use at home on a daily basis. The program makes the user perform all the normal eye movements, including convergence, with the aid of slow- and fast-moving targets and random dot stereograms, which create a 3D image that the child can see when wearing special glasses with red/blue lenses.

Two months later, Lenny had the full range of normal eye movements but was still having some problems with his schooling. Unfortunately, he had a lot of catching up to do and needed to correct mistakes he had learned in the past. However, with his new high level of confidence and a little extra tutoring it was not long before his school reports, for the first time ever, began to glow.

In parallel with the emergence of dyslexia and dyspraxia, there is ADD and ADHD to contend with. These two conditions are an inability to concentrate on the job at hand or an inability to concentrate, combined with a tendency for the individual to cause disruption to his or her environment, due to an inability to remain still for more than a few seconds.

ATTENTION DEFICIT HYPERACTIVE DISORDER (ADHD)

ADHD is not included in any of my medical dictionaries but is included in the *Diagnostic and Statistical Manual of Mental Disorders* (4th edition, known as DSM-IV)—one of the bibles of medical conditions.

This condition is poorly understood and it has been given three distinct subtypes to cover the various forms it may take.

To be diagnosed as ADHD, the symptoms must have been present for more than six months, be inappropriate for the child's age and intelligence, have developed before the age of seven, and have a negative impact in at least two social settings—home and school, for instance. The symptoms of ADHD fall into three main categories—hyperactivity, impulsivity and inattention.

The hyperactivity manifests itself as an inability to sit still, with constant foot tapping and fidgeting, disruptive behavior in the classroom, excessive talking, and an inability to do anything quietly. The child will often act in a silly childish way, is attention-seeking, rough with his and others' toys, and unfortunately often ends up hurting other children.

The impulsivity can be in both communication and actions. The child will attempt to answer the question before it is completed, almost desperate to be the first to answer, or will interrupt a conversation with an inappropriate question. The child cannot wait his turn, intrudes into others' play and tends to have a short fuse and erupts, lashing out, when frustrated.

Though the two conditions overlap, the "inability to pay attention" aspect of ADHD not surprisingly provides an accurate description of what is categorized as ADD. This inattention is seen as: having a poor attention span, making silly mistakes, not completing tasks, not appearing to be listening, being easily distracted, having a poor short-term memory and avoiding anything that involves a sustained mental effort. To complicate things further, ADHD and ADD are often said to coexist.

Children with developmental delay invariably suffer from low self-esteem and this is often present in the child with ADHD symptoms, which should not be missed even though outwardly the child seems fairly robust. The frustration that can lead to violent outburst is a clear sign of the hopelessness many of these children feel but cannot express.

With ADHD, in particular, there is also another very worrying aspect that the parent not only fails to recognize, but unwittingly panders to. Many of these children are carbohydrate addicts, sugar junkies, surviving on a diet high in carbohydrates and little else. Again and again we hear that the child has always been a fussy eater and that the parents have allowed the child to dictate the diet, working on the premise that it is better that they eat something than nothing.

The problem is that the brain's pleasure center loves the sudden influx of sugars, but as the levels begin to fall, craves the next fix. This group of children are often "sugar junkies" and, disturbingly, there is now strong evidence that this addiction can be carried over into adult life, leading to an addiction to alcohol and/or drugs. (Read more about this in Chapter 13.)

How ADHD affects children at school and in later life

Children with symptoms predominantly of ADHD may suffer the same fate as children with dyslexia, as the hyperactivity and poor ability to concentrate will impact upon learning. They, too, often suffer from low self-esteem, get into trouble and live in a world that they cannot understand.

Clearly these children will not get the best from the education that is provided for them, but unfortunately this will also apply to the other children in the classroom as the disruptive behavior and the need for extra supervision by teaching staff to manage the overactive child leaves the others disadvantaged. These children often end up excluded from school and their parents are faced with a struggle to find a school for them.

With regard to the current treatment of ADHD, there is now a body of evidence emerging that would suggest that children who are treated by the standard medications prescribed may well show some signs of improvement in terms of behavior and the ability to concentrate, but at the cost of permanent brain damage. If these claims turn out to be true we must now consider the impact that this will have both at a personal level and in terms of the effects upon society (for more on this, please see Chapter 13).

ATTENTION DEFICIT DISORDER (ADD)

Again, this condition does not appear in any of my medical dictionaries. ADD is a term used to describe a child who has difficulty focusing and maintaining attention. A child must exhibit six or more of the following diagnostic criteria to be considered as suffering from ADD:

1. often fails to pay attention to detail and makes careless mistakes
2. often has difficulty sustaining attention

3. often does not seem to listen
4. often fails to complete work
5. often has problems with organization
6. often avoids/dislikes tasks that involve mental effort
7. often loses things
8. is easily distracted
9. is often forgetful

The child with ADD generally behaves like any other child—misbehaving, being silly and daydreaming—the only difference being the constant and extreme nature of the behavior pattern. When the child's behavior impacts upon family life and schooling, it can be judged to be a problem.

Although inattention or the inability to focus on a particular activity is the hallmark of this supposed condition, the converse can occur, for instance when the child plays a computer game for hours on end. In general the word that perhaps describes ADD best is distractibility. They are distracted by any stimulus in the environment, whether it be color, movement or sound, and almost appear to be looking for anything that will give them cause to look away from the task set before them.

The other aspects often associated with ADD again point to the fact that ADD is a symptom of developmental delay and not a cause in itself. Impulsivity, hyperactivity, clumsiness, mood swings and poor social skills have all been closely associated with ADD. If we were to replace those behavioral traits with known conditions the sentence would read—ADHD and dyspraxia—in fact an underfunctioning prefrontal cortex.

Attention deficit disorder—Thomas, aged nine

Thomas came into the world following a perfect pregnancy and delivery. There was no history of any developmental delay in his family and he met all the developmental milestones months in advance.

*From about seven years of age his parents noticed that Thomas had real **problems concentrating**, a fact borne out by his rather disappointing school reports, and it was not long before the label ADD was firmly attached to him.*

During the consultation process it became very clear that

*Thomas had always been **clumsy**, having had numerous accidents as a consequence, and still had problems attaining **motor skills**. On direct questioning it also became apparent that Thomas liked his little **rituals** and became distressed if any changes were made to his daily routine.*

His medical history included asthma, eczema and recurrent ear infections, during one of which he had experienced a seizure.

Thomas was treated initially by having his diet modified and by being provided with specific exercises. Next he started a short course of treatment at the clinic using the Interactive Metronome. Put simply, this treatment involves the child watching a brief video clip of another child performing a simple exercise, e.g. foot tapping. The child then has to copy the exercise he or she has observed but in strict time with a beat (metronome) generated by the computer. For hand exercises a pad is fitted to the palm of the hand, while exercises involving the feet are carried out using a footpad. Children wear earphones during the treatment session and are informed via various bleeps how accurate they are—very early, early, on time, late or very late— in completing the exercise in time with the metronome beat. This basically retrains the timing mechanisms of the brain and insures, as far as possible, that they are pretty well equal from side to side, meaning that the two sides of the body learn to work in concert.

The response to the treatment for Thomas was little short of miraculous. Within six weeks he had become alert, could concentrate and was unusually attentive to his homework. Feedback from the school was equally pleasing and included comments that Thomas was working well in class, was far more attentive and was now, for the first time ever, both asking and answering questions.

OBSESSIVE-COMPULSIVE DISORDER (OCD)

Obsessive-compulsive disorder is defined as a condition marked by compulsion to perform certain acts repetitively or carry out certain rituals—it is characterized by obsessional traits, and may present simply as a need in the child to place certain objects in a preordained order. At the other extreme it is a condition that can dominate the child's life, where order and routines make normal everyday life unbearable or unlivable.

The adult form of this condition can be severe enough to be

time-consuming, occupying hours of the day and causing marked distress, both mental and physical. Sufferers may, for example, wash their hands so many times that their skin becomes raw.

In childhood the situation may not be so severe but may still occupy a significant amount of the child's day. Washing, checking and ordering rituals are particularly common in children.

When talking to parents it is often difficult to explain to them what is meant by OCD and it is sometimes necessary to give examples. On one occasion, for instance, I cited the activity of arranging every item in the larder by size, type and shape, only to be interrupted by the daughter saying to her anxious mother, "That's *you*!"

Commonly, however, in childhood OCD is subtle and can only be observed during play, for instance when toy cars have to be placed in a particular order, or dressing, when certain items have to be put on first. (Was this Superman's problem with wearing his pants on the outside, or was it just a dressing dyspraxia?)

OCD is often associated with anxiety and depression but is particularly related to Tourette's syndrome.

TOURETTE'S SYNDROME OF CHILDHOOD

Tourette's syndrome is defined as a rare form of generalized tic usually beginning in childhood, between two and fifteen years of age and marked by uncontrolled continuous gestures, facial twitching, foul language and repetition of sentences spoken by other persons. At one time it fell within the purview of the neurologist and was typified by the stereotype of an adult with a severe tic and a habit of letting fly expletives in association with the tic. We've all seen Tourette's portrayed in this way in films, but today we know that this is not necessarily the case. It would appear that more and more children are manifesting tics and subtle signs of Tourette's that might be no more than a frequent clearing of the throat or facial grimacing.

Far from being rare, researchers now consider aspects of tics to be evident in virtually all children at some point in their development as the brain is growing and maturing. Often the signs are so subtle that even parents aren't aware that their child is showing signs of Tourette's along with the more obvious aspects of dyspraxia, ADHD and OCD that may be happening at the same time. These subtle signs may be no more than repeated throat clearing, grunting, blinking or grimacing. But aren't these all signs that parents some-times see in their overtired or anxious child? Yes, the repetition of words or sentences is something we all do as a learning process—it is only when the symptoms increase and persist that concerns should be raised. The use of bad language is part of a caricature of Tourette's and is actually pretty rare. Tourette's syndrome of child-hood is currently said to afflict one child in every hundred.

How Tourette's and OCD will affect the child at school and in later life

A child with OCD or Tourette's syndrome may suffer an almost intolerable daily turmoil, a misery often only shared with a parent, as they struggle with the compulsions that they can in part control but ultimately must give in to. These children not only suffer from low self-esteem but also terrible frustrations and inner sadness often made worse by tactless comments. It is not unusual for these chil-dren to hide themselves away in order to give in to the compulsion that will free them temporarily from the affliction. When confronted by a parent over their behavior the child may react violently or burst into tears, unable to cope with the expectations of others and their own inner conflicts.

Tourette's syndrome—Roland, aged eight

Roland was brought to see me having already been diagnosed as suf-fering from Tourette's syndrome. The family history included OCD and tics on the father's side of the family.

*His birth had been by elective caesarean section at 38 weeks due to a breech presentation. Following the birth Roland had been taken to a special care unit due to concerns over **respiratory distress**. Following this initial hiccup, all milestones were achieved on time or indeed precociously, and all went well until about three years of age. Insidiously, Roland developed the habit of **blinking** for no apparent reason and over the next three years developed a marked **titubation** (a repetitive movement of the body—in this case nodding of the head and rocking to and fro). Gradually he started **grimacing**, repeat-edly **clearing his throat** and exhibiting **echolalia** (repeating the last sentence heard). Added to this there were also **spontaneous move-ments** of both the right arm and leg, lip smacking and licking.*

During the consultation process it also became clear, not

*surprisingly, that he had **learning disabilities**, aspects of **clumsiness**, periods of **obsessive behavior** and an **inability to concentrate** on the matter at hand.*

*Treatment at Tinsley House Clinic involved **afferentating** the left cerebellum by simple peripheral manipulative techniques—professionally manipulating joints in a similar way to how people crack their knuckles. These techniques are sometimes used by chiropractors and osteopaths to treat conditions of the limbs, but here are used to send a barrage of messages to the cerebellar hemisphere on the same side as the manipulated limb. Although not painful it does often mildly shock the individual, particularly the first couple of times. We also demonstrated a set of balancing exercises to be completed daily at home.*

Following his second treatment Roland's mother reported that the titubation, grimacing and involuntary movements of the limbs had dramatically reduced. After two more visits to the clinic, all the tests carried out were clear. Over the next few months all of the signs and symptoms faded away, but Roland's parents were advised to continue with the treatment at home twice a week for the foreseeable future.

AUTISM

So far we have considered dyslexia, dyspraxia, ADD, ADHD and obsessional traits, but what about autism? How does this fit in with this reclassification based on these signs and symptoms forming defined syndromes?

An alternative name for the "autistic spectrum" is pervasive developmental disorder, and this would fit in quite well within my proposed new classification of Development Delay Syndrome. The three key symptoms for autistic spectrum disorders include poor development of social skills, communication and imagination, but may also occur in association with dyslexia, ADD and ADHD.

All the subgroups of autism that have been suggested to date, including Asperger's syndrome, overlap with each other and the boundaries are unclear. It has now been suggested that *true* autism is due to the *absence* of spindle cells. In other words, the spindle cells among the second wave of brain cells that develop four months after birth are either not produced or else they die (see Chapter 4 for more on these cells).

However, in reality if you examine a patient with "typical autism"—that is, a patient with autistic tendencies—you will find aspects of dyspraxia, dyslexia, ADD, ADHD or OCD. If we look at what has been written about the various subgroups of this spectrum we will see that they are merely one end of the entire spectrum of developmental delay syndromes.

Unfortunately, the current *Diagnostic and Statistical Manual of Mental Disorders* (DSM-IV) has lumped together several disorders as being of the autistic spectrum, some of which should be separately classified, as they are definitely not within the developmental delay syndrome spectrum. An example of this would be Rett's disorder, first reported in 1966, which is a genetic disorder characterized by profound mental retardation, reduced skull growth and loss of purposeful hand movements. It has been included under the heading Pervasive Developmental Delay but has a clear, separate genetic cause and should really be classed as a separate genetic disorder.

Hans Asperger published a paper in 1944 in which he described the behavioral characteristics of a group of young boys. It was not until 1994 that Asperger's syndrome was itself added to DSM-IV and therefore considered as a medical condition. Children with Asperger's syndrome can exhibit a variety of characteristic signs and symptoms, and the disorder can range from mild to severe. Already this description is beginning to sound suspect, particularly when we consider the signs and symptoms in a little more detail.

Included in the signs and symptoms of Asperger's syndrome are:

- stilted speech lacking prosody (the lilt or musical quality of speech)
- dyslexia
- dyspraxia
- obsessional traits
- problems reading non-verbal communication

Viewed as a more pronounced form of a developmental delay syndrome, it is easy to see why children initially diagnosed as having ADD or ADHD can be rediagnosed later as having Asperger's syndrome.

The presentation of autism varies widely and many individuals with more severe forms have identifiable underlying medical conditions including a variety of congenital, chromosomal and metabolic diseases. "True" autism occurs when the spindle cells do not develop at all. Because of this, it is not responsive to the form of treatment offered at Tinsley House.

At first glance it would appear that a clear distinction exists between Asperger's syndrome and typical autism based on IQ levels. Initially, one gets the impression that individuals with Asperger's syndrome have average to high IQs, and those with autism have below-average IQs. However, this is not strictly the case and approximately one-third of children with autism have average or above average IQs. If we were to take out of the equation all the conditions that have a definite congenital, chromosomal or metabolic cause, the figures then become far less daunting.

3

THE CONDITIONS REDEFINED

In this chapter we will cover:

- learning and behavioral difficulties as we know them and how they need to be redefined so that we can understand the real causes;
- why the underlying problem that causes dyspraxic, dyslexic, ADHD and ADD symptoms has not been correctly identified until now;
- new insights as to what the problem is and how it can be treated.

LEARNING AND BEHAVIORAL DIFFICULTIES BY ANOTHER NAME

The Learning Disability Myth offers a unique and successful clinical program for treating learning and behavioral difficulties. The treatment is simple, non-invasive and drug-free, and offers a new way of looking at and treating these problems. The differences start right from the beginning in the way that we describe and diagnose learning disabilities, so let's look at these first.

Many people have tried unsuccessfully to find a treatment for learning and behavioral difficulties. At Tinsley House Clinic we now believe that the reason an effective solution has been elusive is that everyone was looking in the wrong place.

As we saw in Chapter 2, the labels commonly used to classify learning and behavioral difficulties are attention deficit hyperactivity disorder (ADHD), attention deficit disorder (ADD), dyslexia, dyspraxia, obsessive-compulsive disorder (OCD), autism and Tourette's.

Before we can propose an effective treatment for learning and behavioral disorders/symptoms, we need to redefine the conditions. (You'll see how it is then easier to look for an underlying cause, a reason why a child has the symptoms they have, and from that new perspective understand what is needed in terms of treatment to remedy the situation.)

At Tinsley House we believe that the labels used to describe learning and behavioral difficulties are not only confusing but of little use or value. We are not the only people who believe this, but we are the first to put forward a logical, scientific argument for why this is so. I have discovered a new way of looking at these symptoms and have accordingly devised an effective treatment program that radically transforms the lives of the children who undergo the treatment.

The most significant reason that the labels are not useful is that *all* of the conditions named above are *symptoms* rather than *conditions*, and they are, in fact, symptoms of a wider underlying problem. It is that underlying problem that we should focus on for treatment rather than simply concentrating on the symptoms.

This is fully explained in the next two chapters but, for now, let's just say that the real problem is a delay in the brain maturing. This immaturity in the brain means that it doesn't function properly, and so we see symptoms of ADHD, ADD, dyslexia etc. At Tinsley House Clinic when we see these symptoms we don't think, "Ah, that child has ADD." We think, "That child has ADD symptoms which means that they have an immaturity in the brain. Let's find out where in the brain and treat it."

So the treatment at Tinsley House Clinic is focused on helping the child's brain to develop properly.

The Learning Disability Myth may well offer the world's first effective solution for learning disabilities. I agree wholeheartedly with those experts who say that dyslexia does not exist, and I would go further and say the same about dyspraxia, ADD, ADHD, OCD and Tourette's syndrome. But what is even more exciting is that I have also discovered, and will reveal in Chapter 4, *when* these problems occur as well as *why* they occur.

I have called all these so-called "conditions" developmental delay syndrome, because on close examination I realized that dyslexia, dyspraxia, ADD, ADHD, OCD and Tourette's syndrome of childhood are not disorders in their own right but just symptoms that always occur together. This is a key part of understanding how these learning and behavioral difficulties can be treated.

Another reason that the labels are not useful is because a child will *always* have more than one condition/symptom. As you read through Chapter 2 you will most probably have noticed that your child displayed characteristics from more than one condition. This is something you will find again when your child is assessed and examined, if it is done correctly. (Unfortunately, with the current way of diagnosing, what happens is that the practitioner tends to see evidence of one condition and fixates upon that, ignoring any other symptoms.)

> *Pigeonholing a child into one condition is not a solution. It is limiting. And it is one of the reasons why a solution has been elusive, until now.*

MORE THAN ONE CONDITION

Let's expand on what I said about all children having more than one symptom. You may have been told that your child has a condition, let's use ADHD as an example. You've been told they have ADHD because that is the symptom that is most strongly present, but your child may also show symptoms of dyslexia and dyspraxia. Similarly, a child labeled dyslexic suffers from dyslexic symptoms, but will also show other symptoms. In fact, there isn't a child on this earth who will have dyslexic, dyspraxic, ADD, ADHD or OCD symptoms alone, despite having one of those labels attached to them.

In reality, when a child is properly assessed and examined, they are found to have a mixture of symptoms including dyslexia, dyspraxia, ADD and OCD. Because they are purely symptoms of an underlying problem, each symptom will vary not only in how much of that symptom is present, but also in how it affects the sufferer. This is not a cause for alarm—it may sound awful if you thought your child just has ADHD to find out that's not the only condition they have, but actually this discovery helps enormously in treating the child.

The important thing here is that the symptoms your child displays, and to what degree they show them, will help a neurologist to pinpoint where in the child's brain the problem lies and therefore where the brain most needs help to function properly. This realization is good news, as it is the first step toward finding an effective treatment.

What we've said here is radically different from other views of learning and behavioral difficulties, so to make it easier to follow our method, here is a step-by-step recap of how we came to this method of diagnosis and treatment at Tinsley House Clinic:

- We understood that the following are symptoms: attention deficit hyperactivity disorder (ADHD), attention deficit disorder (ADD), dyslexia, dyspraxia, obsessive-compulsive disorder (OCD), autism and Tourette's.
- These symptoms alerted us to the fact that there must be an underlying cause of these symptoms.
- We found that the underlying cause is a problem of a particular part of the child's brain being delayed in its development.

The next steps were to:

- reclassify learning and behavioral difficulties (as explained below);
- treat the brain by supporting it (through simple exercises) and nourishing it (with the right food and supplements).

The result of this is that the brain will continue to develop, achieving a permanent treatment.

WHAT WILL HAPPEN IF WE TAKE AWAY THOSE LABELS?

Despite offering an effective treatment for learning disabilities, my work may, in the short term at least, cause some alarm for parents, teachers and health professionals. A lot rides on the current labels.

Not only have people become used to these labels but there are a number of practical reasons for their attachment to them as they stand. The key reason is that the help and support given to the child depends upon the child being labeled. (This support varies according to the type of learning disability, as discussed in Chapter 2.)

The problem with these labels is the way in which they tend to pigeonhole children. It is only human nature to do this, but what if the only available pigeonholes are the wrong ones?

With a diagnosis of dyslexia, for instance, I have yet to meet a child that only has dyslexia—there will always be aspects of dyspraxia, ADD and other problems associated with it. Therefore, by assuming that these problems are actual conditions and putting them into the neat little pigeonholes, we are preventing ourselves from seeing the big picture.

HOW DID WE ARRIVE AT THIS NEW PERSPECTIVE ON LEARNING DISABILITIES?

The work at Tinsley House Clinic focuses on the development of the living brain—how it has evolved since we lived in caves and how it functions. The research we've done has revealed that every one of these so-called conditions is only a symptom and not a distinct condition: we believe that they are all in fact one single condition, a condition we call developmental delay syndrome (DDS).

Through this research we've found that the symptoms your child displays can be pinpointed with accuracy as occurring in a particular part of the brain. In short, we can see where the problem is and we can therefore treat it. There is not a single other existing treatment, apart from that at Tinsley House Clinic, which can offer this accuracy and effectiveness.

The discovery that these learning and behavioral difficulties are all due to one fixable problem may be difficult to grasp initially but provides a far less alarming prospect for treating the problem. We know where the problem lies and treating it becomes within our reach.

> *At Tinsley House Clinic we have identified where the underlying problem lies. Knowing where and what the problem is brings fixing the problem within our reach and a lasting solution becomes a reality.*

FUNCTIONAL NEUROLOGY

To understand the thinking behind this subtle and yet ground-breaking change it is necessary to look at the area we specialize in—functional neurology.

Functional neurology is not based so much on pathology—cutting up dead bodies, so popular in recent detective fiction and in TV dramas—but on physiology and developmental neuroanatomy, which means how the brain functions and copes in everyday situations. Much of the research at Tinsley House Clinic involves looking at the living brain to see how it functions, that is, how it works when we are alive.

The key point here is that we use different parts of our brain for each task that we carry out. And mostly, by studying the living brain, we can pinpoint which part of the brain is used for different activities.

For instance, if we were looking at your brain (assuming that you are a parent or teacher) we would be able to detect which part of it is active when you feel content, looking at a child sleeping peacefully in her bed or working quietly on a task you've set her. Or conversely when you are terrified, when you see she is about to step off the curb and into the path of a speeding car.

View of the Left Side of the Human Brain

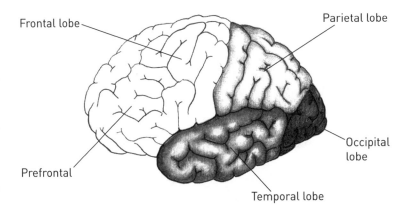

How is this relevant to learning disabilities?

If we know which part of the brain is used for particular tasks, then we can start to make comparisons between how that part of the brain functions when a child is performing a task well and how it functions when the child is having difficulties with a task.

Let's take the example of dyslexia to explain this further. When we first started this work, we asked ourselves the question: what is the child's problem? In the case of dyslexia it might be reading, so let's have a look at what is happening in their brain and how it is functioning when they are trying to read.

By studying the brain, we consistently observed that children with dyslexia always have lower than average activity in the particular area of the brain that takes care of reading. On the other hand, in ADHD you would see higher than average activity in a particular part of the brain that all children with ADHD would show to some extent. If you did a brain scan of children with different conditions, you would see this increased/decreased activity in different areas of the brain.

At Tinsley House Clinic we rely on eye, balance and other examinations to discover which part of the brain is experiencing problems. Locating and observing the area of the brain that is affected in each learning disability are the most revolutionary and exciting aspects of our work.

This link had not been made by anyone before. And, as you can imagine, this has important ramifications for how a child can be treated.

We then considered that if we stimulated the area of the brain that is affected we should see an improvement in the child's ability to do the relevant tasks. The results were very exciting, much more so than we could have imagined.

By further study of the brain, we also realized that the food that children eat has a huge impact on the efficiency of brain function, and so the right diet has to be a key part of the treatment.

This is best illustrated by the example of diaschisis. Diaschisis means a decline in the activity of an area of brain that occurs because of a decline in activity of a functionally related and yet perhaps distant area of the central nervous system. The scientific literature is full of references to diaschisis but the starting point in the understanding of developmental delay syndrome was the description of the cerebellar diaschisis.

Here's an example to explain this more clearly. Let's say your leg is not working properly because you have injured it. This lack of use will have a resulting effect on that part of the brain that controls the function of moving your leg, causing that part of the brain to slow down through lack of use. It follows that if the leg is not working as it should when there is *no* injury then a neurologist will need to test to see if there is a problem with the part of the brain that controls that function.

The cerebellum—literally little brain—lives alone in the back of the skull, below the main part of the brain with only the brain stem for company (see illustration below). Yet it can be considered as the computer that drives the brain itself. If the cerebellum under-functions, then the brain will suffer as a direct consequence, and vice versa.

A LITTLE SCIENCE ABOUT THE BRAIN

The cerebellum, like the brain, is divided into a right and left hemisphere. The right cerebellar hemisphere drives the left cerebral hemisphere and vice versa. Therefore if the left cerebellar hemisphere were to under-function, for whatever reason, then the right cerebral hemisphere would most likely also have problems.

This relationship is fundamental to the proper functioning of the

View of Inside Surface of the Right Hemisphere of the Brain

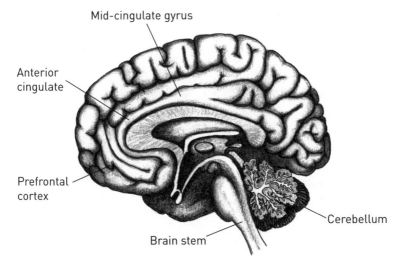

Mid-cingulate gyrus

Anterior
cingulate

Prefrontal
cortex

Cerebellum

Brain stem

brain and has proved to be a stumbling block in some areas of research. Without the knowledge of a second wave of brain cells that develops four months after birth—to be described in Chapter 4—the cerebellum has been wrongly accused of being the site of developmental delays and even autism.

The cerebellum and brain stem share the back of the skull, but also share a very special function. Together they set the basis for temporal sequencing—roughly speaking, setting a time frame in which all motor activity can be set—plus sequencing the motor activities of the two sides of the body.

If there is a problem here due to an aberrant relationship between the cerebellum and brain stem, and the brain, it will produce (to varying degrees) dyspraxic symptoms. If disruption of the cerebellar/brain stem connection can produce symptoms of dyspraxia, it is not a huge step forward to realize that desynchronizing the brain's rhythm would cause numerous problems. These could manifest themselves in many different ways and cause an apparent slowing of the brain's processing speed and thereby functioning.

As mentioned earlier, all of the problems that we see in children with developmental delay symptoms are things we expect to see affecting all children, but to a lesser extent.

Here are some examples that will be familiar to many parents:

- Slow learning to tie shoelaces
- Messy eating
- Accident-prone
- Sloppy dresser

A TYPICAL SCENARIO WITH A DDS CHILD

You're running late and in a hurry to get your child to school. You have repeatedly asked him to put his shoes on, but he seems to be in another world. Eventually, when you resort to shouting, at worst, the "average" child eventually responds. The child with DDS appears "deaf," oblivious, in another world—and they behave like this pretty consistently, not just when preoccupied or tired as with the "average" child.

IF NOT THE CONDITIONS AS WE KNOW THEM, THEN WHAT?

To recap, we must do away with the idea that dyslexia etc. are diseases in their own right. So if they're not conditions and instead they are symptoms, what are they symptoms of? Well, they are symptoms of an underlying problem of immaturity in the brain, particularly involving new brain cells that develop four months after birth (see Chapter 4).

To be clear about where in the brain the problem lies and the symptom patterns this will produce I have suggested four clearly identifiable sub-classifications of the developmental delay syndrome that may help you to grasp this new concept.

A syndrome is a defined collection of signs and symptoms which together form a recognized condition.

This is how we should organize a reclassification of the conditions. (Note: ADD will be prominent in all four types.) The four sub-types of the syndrome named to date are:

1. Developmental delay syndrome—dyslexic type
   When dyslexia is the predominant feature of the child's problem
2. Developmental delay syndrome—cerebellar type
   When dyspraxia is the predominant feature
3. Developmental delay syndrome—Tourette's/OCD/ADHD type
   When tics or obsessive behavior are prominent features
4. Developmental delay syndrome—pervasive type
   When autistic tendencies are present

Treating the individual child is something we do every day at Tinsley House Clinic, but to bring about a global reconceptualization concerning the diagnosis of these worrying difficulties will take a great deal of re-education. To change public opinion and government legislation will take time.

Having redefined these problems, and realized that all of these common learning disabilities are merely symptoms of an underlying immaturity of the brain, we have taken a huge step forward in our understanding of what is happening, but have not yet explained the cause of the underlying malfunction.

To understand why there is this immaturity in human brains that causes the symptoms of dyslexia, dyspraxia, ADHD, ADD, Tourette's and OCD, we will next look at the discovery we've made about some very special cells within the brain that truly define our humanity.

4

WHAT IS GOING ON IN THE BRAIN OF CHILDREN WHO HAVE DDS AND WHY DO THESE SYNDROMES OCCUR?

In the previous chapter I explained that:

- dyslexia, dyspraxia, ADD, ADHD, OCD and tics are not conditions but symptoms;
- they present in a unique way in every child;
- children always have more than one of these symptoms.

Let us recap on the seven key points of a radical new treatment for learning and behavioral difficulties:

1. New research (conducted by Tinsley House Clinic) has allowed for a groundbreaking redefinition of learning disabilities.
2. Dyslexia per se does not exist, nor does dyspraxia, nor ADD nor ADHD, etc. They are very real symptoms, but not conditions.
3. They are symptoms that always appear in patterns, which we call a syndrome.
4. The underlying problem is an immaturity in the brain due to the delayed development of special brain cells that only appear four months after birth.

5. This brain immaturity means that the child's brain cannot cope adequately with everyday tasks and we therefore see symptoms of dyslexia, ADHD, ADD, dyspraxia, etc.
6. The condition that they are suffering from is a developmental delay syndrome, itself due to a delayed maturation in a process called bpoptosis—the name I have given to the missing link in the development of the brain.

So what is it that is happening in the human brain to cause these syndromes? To find the answer we need to look into the evolution of mammals and then consider the developments that have taken place in humans in terms of brain cells growing smarter and more efficient. This is known as "brain specialization."

A LITTLE SCIENTIFIC BACKGROUND

As animals become more complex in their anatomy, and therefore in how they are able to function, they require a more structured nervous system to match this development. This is especially true of certain mammals and birds that have adopted the biped stance—upright, on two legs. Within this group we can include the marsupials, rodents and primates, all of whom can stand on their hind legs, should they want to.

However, of these groups only humans and birds can stand upright all the time. In the case of humans this upright stance has led to some disadvantages (see overleaf) but these have been greatly outweighed by the considerable advantages given by freeing up the arms to do things other than just moving about.

Standing on two legs rather than on four provides greater height, which means that we have a better view of what is around us. From a survival and hunting point of view this is a great advantage. Also, by bringing our eyes in closer together at the front of the head, rather than at the sides, we have been able to obtain stereoscopic vision (this is when each eye has a slightly different picture that the brain then combines to form a single image that also contains *depth*—the third dimension). This has meant that we not only see further due to our increased height, but we are also able to see more clearly and judge such things as the speed and distance of a target object. The disadvantage is that our nose has had to become smaller as the eyes move closer together, and therefore our powers of smell have reduced.

Being able to stand on "hind" legs and use their arms freely also gave our ancestors the opportunity to become toolmakers, and this made them far better hunters as well as survivors. However, standing on two legs does have certain requirements, the most important of which is the ability to defy gravity in order to remain standing. Acquiring the skill to stay upright, as well as becoming more advanced through using our hands, required the growth and development of the nervous system that must receive, process and respond to an ever-increasing workload of sensory data.

NEW BRAIN

To be the human beings we have evolved into today has meant that our brains have had to grow, and new pathways develop so that the new part of the brain can work. This is very like a small town that is growing in size—as it increases and has more shops and services we then need more roads for us to get to them. If we can't get to the shops we can't use them. So it is with the brain; new connections have to be made if new and sophisticated parts of it are to be used.

To do this work, the brain has expanded, developing ever-increasing quantities of neocortex (new brain) overlying the paleo- and archio-cortex (old brain). As the brain is contained within the skull, the skull too has had to evolve and expand in size in order to house and protect the delicate evolving brain tissue.

This is all very well, but we now come up against a problem—namely, that of the bony pelvis and the birth canal in females. There comes a point when, if the brain and therefore the human skull keep on enlarging, they would be too big for the bony birth canal and delivery would prove impossible.

Nature has been attempting to deal with this problem for thousands of years and has come up with various strategies. Neanderthal man, or rather woman, developed an enlarged pelvis that would allow the birth of a child with the larger skull size. Ideally a human child should stay in the womb until at least 21 months, meaning that its brain would be sufficiently mature so that at birth it could soon be walking and on its way to independence. Two problems arise in this situation. First, few mothers would be able to endure such a long gestation period and, secondly, the child would be too big to be delivered. However, the legacy of Nature's attempt to solve the problem with an enlarged pelvis lives on in the female body shape (and that is why women constantly ask "Does my butt look big in this?").

Hence the solution to the problem is to have the child delivered prematurely at nine months, thus greatly extending the necessary nurture period after birth when the child is totally dependent upon the parents.

If we compare a few developmental facts relating to the newborn chimpanzee and the newborn human baby we will see quite clearly how this strategy works. At birth the chimp and human baby both have approximately the same sized brain, but their abilities are very different.

The chimp:

- can walk one month after birth;
- has an adult brain at seven months;
- can lead a relatively independent life and survive alone if need be after seven months.

The human baby:

- cannot walk until about one year;
- does not achieve the full-size adult brain for years—adolescence or later;
- requires an extended period of nurturing if it is to survive.

There is also a difference in terms of the size of their brains at birth and the size they finally grow to. The chimp's brain grows from 350cc at birth to 450cc, whereas the human brain grows from 350cc at birth to 1400cc.

So it would seem that we are not ready to be born at nine months. Our brains are incomplete. Also, while humans have the same size brain as a chimp at birth, our brains grow to be significantly larger. More importantly, there is a difference in the numbers of a certain type of brain cell. One of these types, spindle cells, have been known about for years, but only recently have I discovered their importance in terms of our humanity.

Apart from humans, spindle cells are found only in the brains of animals that we think of as being most like us. They are bonobos (pygmy chimpanzees), chimpanzees, orangutans and gorillas. However, in terms of numbers of spindle cells found in these species, orangutans have only a few spindle cells in their brains; gorillas, chimps and bonobos have increasing numbers, but still not that many. By contrast, humans have tens of thousands of spindle cells.

SPINDLE CELLS MAKE US HUMAN

It is the development of a new wave of cells in the human brain at four months of age that makes us unlike other animals. It is only humans who suffer from learning and behavioral difficulties so it makes sense to look at the brain cells that make us uniquely human. That's where the answer to developmental delay lies, in spindle cells.

It is key to understanding how an immature or incomplete brain can affect our children, that we appreciate that these cells are only to be found in humans and our close ancestors, and that they are only found in a small area of the brain called the prefrontal cortex, the front of the brain. This area of the brain has been implicated in the guiding of attention, pain and fear, and also in modulating the workings of the autonomic nervous system, which controls all the things that we don't think about—heart rate, blood pressure etc.

Clearly the presence of these cells in so few species must have special significance, especially when we consider that in humans, who possess the greatest number of them, there are over 100,000 such cells.

THE FRONT OF THE BRAIN (PREFRONTAL CORTEX)

It is the prefrontal cortex that gives us our humanity, permitting us to live harmoniously in highly structured and regulated societies. It also gives us amazing concepts such as time and thereby the ability to plan events far into the future.

To summarize, humans are unique among living creatures because:

- we stand on two feet most of the time;
- we have an exceptionally well-developed brain;
- we have the largest number of spindle cells in our brains of any species;
- we are born prematurely (that is, not ready to fend for ourselves) by many months.

View of Inside Surface of the Right Hemisphere of the Brain

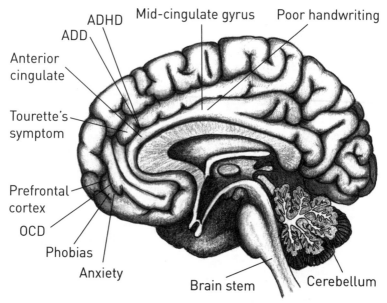

It is our uniqueness as a species that makes us so vulnerable and the only species that suffers from the specific syndromes discussed in this book. Spindle cells are found in the brains of no other animal on the planet except for those of humans and the great apes. Spindle cells develop in the brains of orangutans, gorillas and chimps before they are born. Because we are born prematurely, in humans they only appear four months after birth.

Spindle cells are crucial for us to function as well as we possibly can as human beings. An absence of spindle cells results in autism, while under-functioning spindle cells cause ADD and ADHD. Furthermore, all areas of the prefrontal cortex must work together for us to develop normally.

- Spindle cells are found only in the brains of humans and the great apes. No other animal on the planet has them.
- Spindle cells develop in the brains of orangutans, gorillas and chimps before they are born. In humans they only appear four months after birth.
- Spindle cells are only found in the newest part of the brain— the prefrontal cortex.
- There are more spindle cells in the right side of the brain.
- The right side of the brain is the seat of developmental delay.

If spindle cells survive and function normally then we are equipped with the skills and abilities that make us human. Without the prefrontal cortex and its special cells time would not exist—only day and night.

- The prefrontal cortex allows us memories of the future—in other words we can *plan*.

WHY WE SHOULD BE THE ONLY ANIMALS TO SUFFER FROM DDS CAN BE EXPLAINED SIMPLY BY TAKING IN TWO FACTS

Firstly, being born prematurely and therefore having an immature and incomplete brain makes us vulnerable to any stressor. Stressors can include:

- the level of estrogen in the mother's blood when pregnant;
- fetal distress at birth;
- a diet containing additives and too much salt and sugar;
- a lack of certain essential fats, and nutrients.

We will look at the first two factors below and consider diet and food additives in detail in Chapter 9.

Secondly, the very protective nature of the prolonged nurturing, particularly in a civilized society, means that the infant death rate falls, natural selection is avoided and weak genes can perpetuate. If you happen to be a newborn gazelle with a genetic problem, the chances are you will end up being dinner for the local lion pride. Not so with humans, and so minor genetic problems can go unnoticed and be passed on.

GENETICS—DO THEY PLAY A PART?

The chances of genetic problems being passed on in one or more offspring are in the region of 32 percent if the mother has a defined developmental syndrome, but this rises dramatically to more than 70 percent if it is on the father's side. The fact that one or both parents have had developmental problems does not necessarily mean that their offspring will be affected, but the predisposition will be there.

BIRTH TRAUMA AND FETAL DISTRESS

Our research into the relationship between fetal distress and birth interventions is ongoing but already it is clear that having suffered fetal distress predisposes a genetically susceptible child to developmental delay, as do certain forms of birth interventions. Based on current figures, it would appear that the ventouse delivery has in the past posed a particularly high level of risk.

Fetal distress can be considered as the first warning sign of possible DDS

Unfortunately there is little that we can do about it other than be aware of the risk and make sure that those involved in prenatal care, delivery and postnatal care are well informed of the relationship between birth trauma and developmental delays. Even delaying cutting the cord by a few seconds is now thought to have major implications in terms of development.

I realize that this revelation will be nerve-wracking if you have a child with a developmental delay and are considering having another child. You will probably be eager to know how you can reduce the risks of your subsequent children having a DDS. At this point in time we can't give any clear guidance on how to avoid birth trauma, but it is an area of ongoing research and as soon as new research becomes available we will post it on the Tinsley House Clinic website (www.tinsleyhouseclinic.com).

Finally, in terms of parental expectations, it is essential to realize that intelligence and whatever is happening with these new—second-wave—brain cells are completely separate things. However, the cells that develop at four months of age can impact on the ability of the cells a child is born with to do their job, and therefore they can prevent your child from being as bright as they're capable of.

This is how it works:

1. The first wave of brain cells that develop while you are in the womb give you the potential for intelligence.
2. The second wave of brain cells that develop at four months of age give you the ability to concentrate on what you are doing (to be able to sit still etc.)

The key point here is that even if you are a genius, if you can't concentrate you can't or won't learn properly. A child with developmental delay might appear to be not too bright because they struggle to read and write. Conversely, having their developmental delay treated won't necessarily turn them into a genius: we are what we are.

What having a developmental delay treated will do for your child is that they will improve and progress with their concentration and ability to learn. The right treatment will unleash their full potential and enable them to work toward achieving their goals in life. That surely is good news.

5

FITTING ALL THAT WE KNOW TOGETHER TO FIND A SOLUTION

So far I have explained that:

- we have been wrong to regard dyslexia, dyspraxia, ADD, ADHD, OCD or Tourette's syndrome in childhood as separate distinct disorders;
- they are merely symptoms and signs of an underlying problem;
- these symptoms appear together in varying degrees, unique to every child;
- research at Tinsley House Clinic has redefined them as developmental delay syndromes;
- an effective, non-invasive treatment is now available.

The most exciting part of all this new light on learning and behavioral difficulties is the last one—that at Tinsley House Clinic we offer an effective, lasting and non-invasive treatment.

We must first understand that dyslexia, dyspraxia, ADD, ADHD, OCD or Tourette's syndrome in childhood are symptoms in order to understand how the solution works. They are not what is wrong with your child, they are how the problem—a problem in their not fully developed brain—shows itself.

At Tinsley House Clinic we can locate the problem and do something about it. The parents and children who come here are delighted with the results. This program is available to you in this book—from Chapter 6 onwards.

Your child will need to be properly diagnosed for a full treatment program to be prescribed. At the time of writing, I am the only person who offers this program of treatment but I am hoping that others will be able to offer it soon in the United States and internationally (see www.tinsleyhouseclinic.com for news on that front). What can be done today by using this book is to get started on the Tinsley House Eating Plan (Chapter 11) and to work on your child's behavior with the Parental Survival Plan (Chapter 12). Understanding and learning more about what really causes learning and behavioral difficulties will help enormously and you will know that a solution is possible.

HOW TO FIND A SOLUTION THAT WORKS BY RETHINKING THE CURRENT VIEW OF THE PROBLEM

To find a solution, we must look at the clinical manifestations—that is, how they appear in the child—of the disorders and relate these to the underlying problems in the child's brain. (Exactly how this is done is covered in Chapters 7 and 8 on assessment and examination.)

What this means is that different areas of the central nervous system under-function (we explain the reasons in Chapter 4) and as a result produce signs and symptoms that are commonly called dyslexia, dyspraxia, ADD, ADHD, OCD or Tourette's syndrome in childhood to varying degrees of severity. No two children will have exactly the same problems and therefore can only be diagnosed based on their unique mix of symptoms. Children cannot be properly diagnosed by labeling them and then treating them only based on their main symptom.

When we recognize that the problems experienced by a child who has developmental delay syndrome are so varied it makes perfect sense to forget the old labels and to redefine the way we label and diagnose children. The outcome is an effective, permanent treatment that gets to the root of the problem.

It is the dominance of a particular sign or symptom within a syndrome that often guides the practitioner toward the wrong diagnosis. I have yet to meet a child with only a single symptom and it is for this reason that it is so important to realize that a symptom is not a disorder. Regarding the predominant symptom as a condition in itself limits thinking around what the answer to the problem is. If you're only aware of part of the problem it will be difficult to find a solution.

Let's now look at what has been attempted in terms of treatment and why such treatments don't work.

Looking in the wrong place

In order to treat any condition you have to know just what is causing it. For example, if you have a headache, it could be because you enjoyed yourself, indulging in a little too much to drink the night before, or it could mean that you are having an intracranial bleed. In the first scenario an aspirin might be all you need, while in the second an aspirin could prove disastrous.

> *A headache is a symptom of an underlying problem such as a hangover or a brain tumor. We don't say, "Ah, headache, that's a condition" and leave it at that. If it persists, we investigate further to find the cause.*

For years people have been looking for the cause of dyslexia, but because they considered dyslexia a condition in its own right they were looking in the wrong place. Endless papers have been published noting differences in sizes of various brain structures and numerous theories have been put forward, many sub-classifying dyslexia almost as though they were trying to get the condition to fit the theory. Similarly, geneticists have been trying to find a dyslexia gene. How can they when dyslexia, as a condition, does not exist? It is like looking for a tummy-ache or headache gene when they are just symptoms of something else altogether.

AMAZING FACTS

The prefrontal cortex—otherwise known as the very front of the brain
It is this very front part of the brain that makes us human. Without a mature prefrontal cortex we lack social graces. The very front of the brain—the prefrontal cortex—is basically three-sided. The symptoms of ADD, ADHD, OCD, panic attacks and anxiety occur when the three sides are not working in harmony. The front of the brain continues to develop until we are eighteen years of age.

Which part of the brain does what?
The very front of the brain allows us memories of the future—that is, the ability to plan ahead and remember those plans.

Fifty-seven percent of children with developmental delay cannot bring their eyes in toward the nose and therefore have problems reading.

Ninety-eight percent of children with learning and/or behavioral difficulties have a delayed maturation of the right brain.

The discovery of new cell development at four months of age
At birth the human brain is not complete. The human brain contains special brain cells that develop four months after birth that allow us to write, paint etc. Only humans have special brain cells that develop after the brain has formed.

Treatments for dyslexia tend to fall into three distinct types. First, there are a variety of exercises that are prescribed. Then there are devices thought to help limit the visual problems associated with the condition. As well as these, there are educational strategies designed to help the child progress despite their affliction.

One particular exercise program was apparently based on a treatment regime that NASA had to come up with to combat dyslexic symptoms experienced by astronauts after being exposed to weightless conditions for a time. Although the treatment apparently worked for the astronauts, we must bear in mind that the astronauts were adult and the dyslexia only became apparent in conditions of weightlessness, so there is already an enormous difference between them and a child with learning disabilities.

Providing exercises to children with dyslexia that are specifically designed to stimulate the back part of the brain—the cerebellum—will most certainly help at first. However, without a clear understanding of what dyslexia is and what causes it—which leads to applying the correct treatment—they are bound to fail in the long run.

Similarly, providing glasses with colored lenses or putting colored overlays over the page will help (the theory behind this is that it makes it easier for the brain to process the input and reduce the contrast between black and white) but they certainly will not be a permanent solution. In a recent study it was found that 57 percent of children with developmental delay could not bring their eyes in toward the nose when viewing an object close up. If this problem is not addressed then it does not matter what you do in terms of colored filters.

Dyspraxia as a diagnosis is relatively new and very poorly understood by parents and professionals. Again, treatments are based on exercises, which will help to some extent but cannot be a solution to the problem as dyspraxia is never found on its own; there will always be other problems too. Therefore, as with dyslexia, you have to treat the underlying cause, not just one of its signs.

ADHD has been treated by a variety of approaches varying from behavior management to diet, but ultimately vast numbers of children are managed by drug therapy. This can be remarkably effective and the answer to the prayer of parents who are at their wits' end, but controlling the child's behavior using these drugs has come at a terrible cost. Evidence is now emerging that the use of drugs in the management of ADHD causes long-term brain damage. (Notice I did not say treatment, because it is not a treatment—it only manages the ADHD.)

Tourette's syndrome and obsessive-compulsive disorder are so common in childhood as to be considered a "normal" stage that nearly all children pass through. Clearly it is the degree of grimacing or indulging in rituals that is critical here. These signs and symptoms are caused by delays, by degree, in the maturation and functioning of various areas of the brain. If detected early enough they can be treated effectively and will, like the trivial signs observed in virtually every child, gradually fade away. However, unless we recognize the true situation—that is, the delay that can occur in the development of the brain that takes place four months after birth—then these early signs may be missed or mistreated. Again, any drug therapy offered will only manage the condition.

Hopefully, with the breakthrough made at Tinsley House Clinic as to the underlying cause and the understanding that these conditions are no more than symptoms, treatments can now be directed toward the real problem.

At Tinsley House Clinic we have added together what was known and the discoveries I have made to offer a revolutionary new treatment for learning and behavioral difficulties. Some treatments have been close to realizing that the problem lies in the brain, but because no one was looking in the right place they only got part of the way there. What works at the clinic is a bit like how you make a cake, that is, by combining the right ingredients, and putting them together in the correct way so that they work. The ingredients of the Tinsley House treatment are beautifully simple: a brain-supporting (as opposed to harming) diet and simple yet effective brain and eye stimulation exercises.

The question remains: why do these symptoms appear in the first place? We said earlier that Nature has had to come up with certain strategies to get round the problem of fitting a bigger, more sophisticated brain and skull through the birth canal. The answer is to have the baby born prematurely (at nine months rather than 21 months, when the brain would be better developed) and then greatly extend the nurturing period until the child can survive unaided.

> *The human baby at birth is undeveloped both in terms of growth and maturity.*

Part of this growth and development, necessary for the child to become more independent, involves the growth and expansion of the new brain, the very reason the brain is bigger in the first place and hence needs birthing strategies. Although the primitive brain is able to function, it takes time for the neocortex (new brain) to mature and then, and only then, exert a higher level of control over the older, primitive brain.

It is the variability in this process of maturation of the neocortex—some taking longer than others—that generates the various symptoms of developmental delay. Without treatment these symptoms can persist for a lifetime. That is, to some degree or another we will all demonstrate minor symptoms of developmental delay, but as the brain matures and the various areas catch up and level out in terms of function, these symptoms should disappear. However, if there is a genetic predisposition toward a developmental delay and this predisposition is brought into being by fetal distress then the symptoms of developmental delay will appear and remain unless treated correctly.

A prime example of the varying maturity of the brain is in gaining control of the bladder. We all expect babies to have to wear diapers, but at around two years would hope that the child had gained control of their bladder by day and, a little later, at night. There may be the occasional accident—if they've had a big drink before bed or won't get out of bed to go to the toilet because they are convinced that monsters lurk under the bed—but mostly they should be dry.

In terms of gaining bladder control, the frontal cortex has to develop and mature to a point when it can exert control over the more primitive regions of the nervous system, and this development and maturity will vary from child to child, depending upon the various factors we have considered already.

The reason why night control comes after daytime continence is that at night the level of brain activity drops and so there is in effect less control; only when the brain has matured still further and the level of brain activity during sleep is sufficient, can a decision—to pee or not to pee—be made. Bladder control is a developmental milestone, so late control of bladder function can be used as an indication of the level of maturity of the developing brain.

Bladder control is a fairly basic function, so what about the control of the emotions and the development of the social graces?

Let us consider two similar situations with very different outcomes. In the first situation an adult wants to purchase a relatively expensive item and consults with their partner concerning the matter as it involves their joint incomes. The other partner agrees that the purchase would be a good idea but suggests deferring the purchase for a month, by which time the bank balance should be a little healthier. This is agreed and both partners are happy.

In the second situation a young child sees a doll and decides she wants it and wants it right now. The mother explains to the child that she can't afford the doll this week but may be able to buy it at the end of the month. The result is a tantrum and neither mother nor child is happy.

There is an important difference between these two situations. In the first scenario the partner who could not have the object of their desire immediately had a mature adult brain and could cope with what is called "deferred gratification." In other words, you don't get it immediately, you have to wait for what you want. In the second scenario the child could not cope with this deferred gratification and the mother had to suffer the child's tantrum in the middle of the store while other shoppers looked on.

The basic problem here is time. In order to understand that you will get the doll, but not now, you require an understanding of words that relate to time—tomorrow, next week, soon. So to have any chance of understanding time you need to have a well-functioning prefrontal cortex.

With all young children we expect problems like the one mentioned above—it is a normal part of growing up—but what if this were to continue well past the toddler stage? Now you have a real problem. Again this is a clear sign that a part of the prefrontal cortex (the very front of the brain) is delayed in its development. If you read the following case study about Matt, you will see the other parts of the puzzle beginning to fit into place.

A toddler in big-boy's clothing—Matt, aged four and a half

Matt's mother brought him to see me because she was at the end of her rope. In fact she told me later that she had considered taking her own life. She had met Matt's father, fallen in love, married and very shortly had become pregnant with their first child. Helen had been and still was the perfect child, and so when she had fallen pregnant for the second time she had assumed that her second child would be just like his big sister.

The pregnancy, labor and delivery had gone like clockwork until the final stages, when Matt needed a little assistance on entering the world. There had been some concern about his heart rate and a **forceps-assisted delivery** *was performed. Following this minor* *hiccup all had gone well until Matt mastered the all-important skill of walking. From that point on he became a nightmare, always **bumping into things**, always on the move and if ever frustrated— as frequently he was—a tantrum to end all tantrums ensued.*

Before Matt was two his parents had separated, his father apparently unable to cope with the fact that his wife was, more often than not, busy with the children, which left him feeling left out and unloved. Since that time Matt's behavior had deteriorated to the point that his mother felt she could not take him anywhere. Having tried him at nursery school a couple of times she could not face the embarrassment of trying to get him from the car to the school.

While we talked, Matt was systematically wrecking the examining room. Chairs were being tipped over, instruments thrown on the floor and books pulled from the shelves. I was watching Matt out of the corner of my eye but, more importantly, he was watching me, glancing in my direction after each act of vandalism. Having observed, it was time to act. I looked directly at Matt and waited until we had eye contact before asking him to come and sit on the stool in front of me. He considered my request for a split second and then turned away and continued with what he was doing.

At this point I got up and went over to where he was about to shuffle a manuscript and, kneeling down, I moved in toward his face, making direct eye contact and invading his private space. I then told him that he was behaving very badly and that in this room he had to behave at all times. I asked him if he understood. He turned his head away from me to avoid my gaze and was about to continue vandalizing my manuscript when I repeated my question. This time he nodded. I then told him to put the chairs back where they should be and pick everything up off the floor. Reluctantly he responded, but every time he replaced an item he tested me by not doing it as it should have been done. The stool he had knocked over was put where it should be but upside down, etc.

I have to say the consultation/examination was not the easiest; however, the outcome was. Matt showed all the signs of a minor developmental delay but the major problem was, I felt, his behavior patterns and the responses to them from his mother and his very tolerant grandmother. I therefore decided to invite his mother back without Matt so that we could put in place a Parental Survival Plan. Following this meeting I was not at all sure that Matt's mother was convinced that my plan would work, and when she did not call as arranged I was very disappointed. Two days later, though, a very pleased mother called me. Not only was the plan working, but it had been far easier to implement than she had thought and Matt seemed almost pleased to have his temper brought under control.

Once Matt had been controlled his treatment for his developmental delay could begin. After discussion with his mother we had decided that he needed a much healthier diet supplemented by omega-3 and omega-6, and started him on a simple set of exercises designed to get his cerebellum working better. In his particular case this simply involved a balancing exercise while walking up and down the bottom of the stairs and while cleaning his teeth. Later I introduced a computer program, which at varying levels of complexity, helps the child to concentrate on various things—pictures, letters, numbers, symbols—thereby stimulating certain areas of the brain. Virtually from day one Matt has never looked back and my office has remained just as I like it.

IDENTIFYING WHERE AND WHAT HAPPENS IN THE BRAIN

Neurologists have studied the prefrontal lobe and subdivided it into regions, and certain functions have been pinned down as being controlled by particular regions of the brain. The scientific names of these various regions—orbitofrontal, dorsolateral, anterior cingulated etc.—are not important here, as long as we appreciate that it is critical in terms of development delay to realize how such delay will generate symptoms and signs that we may wrongly attribute to a single condition e.g. dyslexia.

Delayed maturation of the very front of the brain is a cause of developmental delay syndromes.

Now that we have grasped the concept of delayed maturation of the neocortex as a cause of developmental delay syndromes, themselves due to various stresses the developing brain may be subject to, we must address the issue of diaschisis.

A diaschisis is defined as a physiological decline in activity in a functionally related but distant part of the brain. What this means is that, if in a normal situation A talks to B and B talks to C, if A or B under-functions then, if C doesn't have any other input, it will also decline in function even though it is nowhere near either A or B.

In the human brain the two cerebellar hemispheres are in communication with the opposite cerebral hemispheres, that is, the right cerebellar hemisphere is in contact with the left cerebral hemisphere and vice versa. Therefore a decline in activity or maturation of, say, one cerebral hemisphere will cause problems functionally with the opposite cerebellar hemisphere. Often the cerebellar symptoms are so pronounced that some scientists have wrongly thought that the cerebellum is the seat of the problem. What in fact we are dealing with is a developmental delay syndrome in which the cerebellar signs predominate due to a diaschisis, thereby overshadowing the symptoms generated by the cerebral hemispheres.

As if this isn't complicated enough, we must also consider the

A View of the Left Half of the Brain stem and Cerebellum

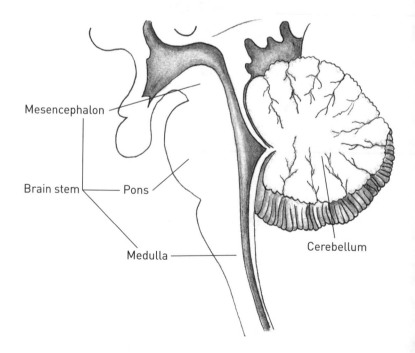

Mesencephalon

Brain stem — Pons

Medulla

Cerebellum

intimate relationships between the cerebellar hemispheres on each side and the brain stem. Put simply, a triangular circuit fires from the bottom of the brain stem to the cerebellum to the top of the brain stem then back down to the bottom again.

This circuit fires at between 8Hz and 12Hz and is thought to function in the timing of movement by literally turning the motor system on and off. Clearly the two sides of the body need to be synchronized and this requires the twin circuits to be firing in a synchronized manner.

It is postulated that if the cerebellum on one side is underfunctioning, or indeed if there is a problem in the brain stem, then the twin circuits are thrown out of synchronicity and dyspraxia, dysmetria or dysdiadochokinesia results.

Dyspraxia is defined as an inability to perform a learned movement accurately.

Dysmetria is an inability to stop a muscular movement at a desired point and is usually described as an undershoot or overshoot.

Dysdiadochokinesia is an inability to make alternating movements in rapid succession, such as turning the palm of the hand up and then down. It is usual to compare the movements of both limbs while performing such a task.

We look for these signs of malfunctioning in our assessment of children to build up a clinical picture of the extent of developmental delay and its severity. We will consider the significance of these signs and others when we look at the examination of the child.

> *Nature's ploy to deliver the baby prematurely gets round the problem of the size differential between birth canal and skull but leaves the child vulnerable, as it is underdeveloped and requires extensive nurturing.*

GENETIC CAUSES/PREDISPOSITION FOR DEVELOPMENTAL DELAY

As we've seen, delivering the baby prematurely gets round the problem of the size differential between birth canal and skull but leaves the child vulnerable, as it is underdeveloped and requires extensive nurturing, and it also creates another potential problem in terms of genetics.

Let's look back to the gazelle example used earlier. If it does not get to its feet soon after birth, it will quite likely be eaten by the local lion pride. In this way Nature insures survival of the fittest and culls out any weaknesses. Our extended nurture period bypasses this cruel fact of Nature. Not only do we have an extended period of nurturing, but that nurturing takes place mostly within the safety of the home and confines of a regulated society, which means that, thankfully, our babies aren't likely to be gobbled up by lions or other similar dangerous beasts despite how long they take to learn to walk. The progress of medicine also means that children don't die from many of the conditions that would have killed them in the past.

It doesn't matter to our survival in the same way as other animals as we are largely protected from death in ways that no other animal is. This is a desirable thing for us humans; the only drawback of both strong and weak being protected alike is that this potentially allows genetic weaknesses to be perpetuated.

So do genetics play a part in the generation or perpetuation of developmental delay syndromes? Unfortunately, the answer is yes. As we have already seen, if there is a history of any type of developmental delay on the mother's side then there is a 30 percent plus chance of one or more of the children developing a delay syndrome. Should the history be on the father's side then the percentage probability shoots up to 70 percent plus. Bear in mind that these figures are probabilities and do not mean that the children of parents with a history of developmental delay will *necessarily* have problems. The figures may be even higher, as we can't be sure whether or not parents have a problem too; often the symptoms may be subtle or well hidden, even from that person themself, or the parents deny any history of such problems.

BOYS AT RISK

Could there be other causes of developmental delay other than genetics? A clue to the answer to this came from looking at the gender bias occurring in developmental delay syndromes. The vast majority (70 percent) of sufferers of developmental delay are boys. As we've discussed earlier the cell development that takes place at four months can be delayed by genetic factors that come into play. Boys are more susceptible to these genetic weaknesses becoming active and the cell development being delayed, as they are more vulnerable to their mother's stress levels when developing in the womb.

It is thought that the male brain is vulnerable to the mother's estrogen level and that if her circulating level of estrogen rises it may affect a developing male brain while a developing female brain remains unaffected. The circulating estrogen level can only have an effect during a critical period of development. However, the fact remains that male brains are more vulnerable during development and remain so during the maturation process.

Also, although the female brain is smaller than the male brain it is now known that certain critical areas of the female brain have a greater surface area and therefore greater functional capabilities. It is claimed that, due to this, the female brain is better suited to cope with the stresses of modern-day living, having greater endurance, coping strategies and multi-tasking capabilities.

HOW CAN WE LIMIT THE FACTORS INVOLVED IN DDS?

So far we have looked at the various reasons why developmental delay syndromes can occur and it is clear that the premature birth strategy devised by Nature provides the underlying predisposition—this is not preventable. Stress factors in the womb play a role, and these may be preventable if we identify how to avoid this happening. Furthermore, the effects of birth intervention may be preventable depending on what can be done to change birthing practices. Genetics, to a degree, throws the final dice, and this may be preventable if future research shows which gene or genes are involved.

Given that these things are unavoidable at this current time our focus should be on being aware of them and discovering if there is anything we can do to limit either the onset or the effect once established.

I have mentioned the importance of good nutrition for children and this has to be the starting point either in "prevention" or treatment. In fact, regardless of whether there is a developmental problem or not, the growing brain needs certain essential elements in the diet, not just to function but to grow, develop and fulfill its potential.

In the next three chapters I will outline the Tinsley House treatment plan, including an explanation of exercises for each symptom, and then describe the assessment and examination process. I will describe foods—good and bad—followed by an eating plan to help you to provide the best possible diet for your child. This treatment has proven startlingly effective in my clinic and, if followed correctly, can also deliver amazing results for your child too.

6

THE TINSLEY HOUSE TREATMENT PLAN

The main purpose of this book is to provide an effective treatment plan for developmental delay syndrome. We have arrived at this new and effective treatment by first redefining the conditions (see Chapter 3) and we now understand that all of the conditions we know as learning disabilities are simply symptoms of a developmental delay.

The good news here is that this makes the problem easier to understand and the search for the cause of the symptoms simpler. As soon as I understood that the problem was that a part or parts of the brain were under-functioning, the treatment needed to remedy the problem—making that part or parts of the brain function better or to their optimum—was clear as day.

The purpose of this chapter is to point out that you are not alone and something can be done. Your child's school can help by providing extra or one-on-one tutoring; you can help your child by providing the right food and supplements. And getting the right assessment and examination at the start, which will determine the treatment, is crucial.

Everyone who reads this book can put their child on the Eating Plan immediately. All children will benefit from a diet free from bad things and instead have a diet packed with beneficial foods. Therefore the food plan will be the same for most children—perhaps stricter for some, depending on their problem, but essentially the same. Of course every child will need to be individually assessed and have a tailored treatment plan, but I will outline how the diagnosis is best made and what the treatment might comprise.

The treatment plan includes:

- assessment (see Chapter 7);
- examination (see Chapter 8);
- a new eating plan (see Chapters 9–11).

Before we go into the treatment plan, let's just recap what we can expect of the "average child." If this isn't your child's experience, then be reassured that this book can help you to help your child to achieve these things and more, fulfilling their potential, unlimited by a learning or behavioral difficulty.

To state what is to be expected of an "average" child would require a full text. However, if we look at the various stages the "average" child will go through and when, clues will begin to emerge that things might not be as they should be.

Important note: all children will differ in their development, some will be faster, some slower, so this should simply be regarded as a guide for the "average" child, and nothing more. There is no need to worry if you find that for any reason your child's behavior does not conform to any of these stages. This is not intended to be a set of hard and fast rules, but merely as broad indications of what you might expect to find.

1. The "average" child may be sitting unaided at six months, crawl (not bottom-shuffle) and be walking at a year.
2. The "average" child may have a collection of single words in the first year, two words together in the second year and be making mini-sentences by the third year.
3. The "average" child may be dry by day at around two and a half years and dry by night shortly afterwards. Bed-wetting incidents may occur but are unlikely to persist, and soiling may not occur.
4. During the first few months of life the primitive reflexes may be replaced by the adult responses. Retained reflexes, e.g. the Babinski sign (see Chapter 8), provide an early clue.

5. The "average" child may daydream and may have imaginary friends, rituals, obsessions or habits.

6. The "average" child may well grimace or blink, particularly when tired, but won't do it regularly.

7. The "average" child will show varying rates of development. Some kids go through a clumsy stage, others are late tying their shoelaces. Some will excel at spelling while others struggle.

The "average" child can be late or struggle with a few of the above but when one or more stages are late from each of the developmental milestones (1–4) and incoordination or behavior is excessive (5–7) there may be cause for concern.

COMMON QUESTIONS ASKED BY PARENTS

This may answer some questions you have before you go to the assessment, or it may remind you that there are other things you'd like to ask.

Q. What is dyspraxia?

A. An inability to perform coordinated and particularly learned movements correctly.

Q. Is my child dyslexic?

A. Possibly, but probably dyspraxic as well with a touch of ADD etc., as these are only symptoms and symptoms that never appear in isolation.

Q. Is it our fault?

A. Definitely not.

Q. Am I a bad mother?

A. I doubt it, but some helpful advice won't hurt.

Q. Does diet make a difference?

A. Definitely, yes.

Q. Will fish oils help?

A. Yes. In fact I would suggest that every child in the land should take omega-3 and omega-6.

Q. What are omega-3 and omega-6?

A. They are essential fatty acids. They are called "essential" as your body and particularly your brain must have them.

Q. Should I have my child put on Ritalin®?

A. No. Read what I have to say first.

Q. What are the side effects of Ritalin®?

A. The minor side effects include loss of appetite and sleep. However, recent research has suggested long-term brain damage and sudden deaths have been attributed to taking methylphenidate (Ritalin®).

Q. Will exercises help?

A. Specific exercises help initially but other treatments are necessary thereafter.

Q. Was it something I did during the pregnancy?

A. No, unless you did something very foolish—with alcohol or drugs—you have nothing to blame yourself for.

Q. Is it genetic?

A. Probably—72 percent of the children attending my clinic have parents with similar learning/behavioral problems.

Q. Can aspartame affect children's behavior?

A. Yes. See what I have to say about it in Chapter 9.

Q. Will my younger children develop it?

A. Not necessarily. That any child will have a developmental delay is only a probability and never a certainty.

Q. Is this mainly a problem with boys?

A. Yes.

Q. Should we take a behavioral management course?

A. Why not try the Parental Survival Plan in Chapter 12 first. If all else fails it might be worth considering if you feel you have totally lost control.

Q. Is too much sugar a bad thing?

A. Yes. See Chapter 9 for more information.

Q. Will he grow out of it?

A. If there is just a tiny problem, then yes, he might. However, if it is a real developmental delay, without treatment, it will be carried over into adult life.

Q. Will the Tourette's get worse?

A. Not necessarily. If treated early on it will respond to the right treatment.

Q. Can dyslexia be permanently treated?

A. Yes. That is why you should read this book.

Q. Will my ADHD son become a criminal?

A. Unfortunately, many children with ADHD do get themselves into trouble and this is why I advocate early treatment.

Q. Can a difficult birth cause problems?

A. Recent research at my clinic would suggest the answer is yes.

Q. Are food additives really a problem?

A. The bad food additives certainly are. See Chapter 9 for more information.

Q. Is it safe to have my child vaccinated with the MMR vaccine?

A. I wish I had the answer to this one but I am afraid I don't. Certain children may be susceptible and react adversely.

OTHER COMMONLY ASKED QUESTIONS AND ANSWERS

My husband and I are both dyslexic. If we have children will they be dyslexic?

A "dyslexia gene" as such has not been identified; therefore the evidence is a little vague. The problem is, I believe, that the geneticists have been looking for a "dyslexia" gene when what they should be looking for is the genes that control the second wave of brain cells that develop after birth. However, what we can say is that if the mother is dyslexic there is a 30 percent chance of one or more of the offspring being dyslexic and if the father is dyslexic the probability rises to 70 percent. In a recent study we conducted at my clinic, 72 percent of the parents of children attending the clinic for learning/behavioral problems stated that they had suffered similar problems.

Our son is seven years old and still wets the bed. Why is this?

The part of the brain that controls the bladder is in the front part on the inside surface. Until this area matures it cannot control the bladder as it should, so when it fills up, it empties. Normally children become dry by day at around two and a half years old and dry at night a little later on. If the brain is a little slow developing, although it can cope by day when the brain is awake, when the brain goes to sleep so does the control center, and you end up with another wet bed. If the brain can be helped to develop normally, bed-wetting stops within a matter of weeks.

What is dyspraxia?

Dyspraxia is what used to be called the clumsy child syndrome. That is, the child with dyspraxia has problems with gross and/or fine motor skills. Dyspraxia can take on many forms and may be evident when the child is dressing, tying shoelaces, feeding, trying to ride a bike or playing sports. In a recent study (Tinsley House, December 2005) it was shown that it never occurs on its own, always forming part of the collection of symptoms of a developmental delay.

Can diet affect my child's behavior?

Yes. The developing brain needs the right building blocks and the right fuel in the right quantities. Modern research has shown that in societies all over the world our diets do not contain many of the nutrients we need and no more clearly is this true than with omega-3. Many studies have shown that the modern diet provides only half of the omega-3 we need. It has been estimated that 60 percent of our brain relies on the essential fatty acids—omega-3 and omega-6—to function, and essential fatty acid deficiency has been implicated in the occurrence of Alzheimer's disease.

Artificial sweeteners have been said to cause glutamate storms, the triggering of abnormal brain activity. The bad food additives have a similar effect, triggering hyperactivity and emotional outburst. Too much sugar can trigger hyperactivity and, more worryingly, has been linked to addiction.

Can my child be treated?

The process that underlies developmental delay is now better understood, and as long as the brain cells that should develop four months after birth are in place, then the answer is yes. However, the child will have to undergo treatment over a variable period of time and the parents may need to address their parenting skills.

What can I do to help?

Monitor your child's diet carefully. Avoid all junk food, bad fats, bad food additives, artificial sweeteners and foods or drinks with high sugar contents. Add omega-3 and omega-6 to their diet at the recommended dosage (see Chapter 10 for more on this).

Demand that food manufacturers stop producing junk for profit and complain on a daily basis to the supermarkets and shops that offer it.

When you have read this book through carefully, seek the appropriate treatment.

Can the school help?

Yes. Speak to the school, particularly your child's teacher/tutor and the person in charge of the school's special education program. They will be able to tell you what the school can offer in terms of one-to-one teaching, extra time for exams, etc.

Does being dyslexic mean my child has a low IQ?

No, it certainly does not. Your child's intelligence is quite separate from their current ability to learn. Once any developmental delay has been addressed your child will attain their full potential.

HOW THINGS COULD CHANGE AT THE SCHOOL LEVEL

In 2005 I was approached by a school that asked if I could provide a screening test for DDS for their children. I thought this an excellent idea, as the sooner problems are detected, the sooner they can be remedied, and this would provide an excellent opportunity for a pilot study. Experience has shown me that the earlier treatment is started—that is, the younger the child—the sooner the treatment takes hold and makes a difference to the child.

Not only does this mean that the child is helped sooner, but also that the child does not have to suffer prolonged bouts of middle ear infections, all the anxiety associated with asthma or the annoyance of eczema—and they are not falling behind at school.

Thus early treatment removes a huge burden from the health service in terms of reduced visits to the doctor and ENT department. It also liberates educational funding for special education and potentially reduces the impact of disruptive children in the classroom.

The screening process is divided up into three parts. Firstly, the parents complete a simple questionnaire designed to detect any genetic trait, known stressing factors and early signs that things might be going wrong.

PARENT'S QUESTIONNAIRE—NAME OF CHILD ....

(a) Is there a family history of any behavioral/learning problems? YES/NO

(b) Was your child premature? YES/NO

(c) Was the birth natural? YES/NO

(d) Did your child suffer fetal distress? YES/NO

(e) When did your child sit unaided? ....months

(f) Did your child crawl? YES/NO

(g) At what age did your child walk? ....months

(h) When was your child dry by day? ....months

(i) When was your child dry by night? ....months

(j) Do you have any concerns about your child? YES/NO

If YES please write a short summary of your concerns below:

Secondly the school completes a questionnaire based on the child's behavior and achievements within the classroom setting.

SCHOOL QUESTIONNAIRE—NAME OF CHILD ....

(a) Are there any behavioral issues/concerns? YES/NO
     If YES please provide a brief summary below:

(b) Are there any learning disabilities? YES/NO
     If YES please provide a brief summary below:

Thirdly, a mini-assessment is given that with the questionnaires will provide a very good idea of what is happening in terms of brain development and maturation. More details are given in Chapter 7.

MINI-EXAM

This includes:

1. Eye tests for visual acuity and convergence
2. Hearing tests
3. Simple tests for cerebellar function

The parents of children identified during the screening assessment would be informed by the school/trust liaison officer of their child's difficulties and would then be given an opportunity to make an appointment for a full assessment at Tinsley House Clinic.

Please note that at the time of writing this book the Tinsley House Clinic is the only clinic that offers the treatments explained in this book, but I am hoping that further clinics will take up my offer to teach them the treatments. We are also planning to set up clinics in the USA and internationally, and I will keep my website up to date with any news on this.

The case below illustrates so many of the things that I have been attempting to get across in this book.

SAM'S STORY—A LETTER FROM HIS ADOPTIVE MOTHER

Pete and I adopted Sam when he was two years old. His birth mother abused herself with drinks and drugs during pregnancy, and he had been moved to foster care at birth. We were told of possible problems with eyesight and hearing and he was already seeing specialists for these problems when adopted by us.

Sam is now seven years old. He has always been an extremely happy little boy and full of fun and energy. He was discharged from the hospital regarding his hearing and eyesight when four years old. His eyesight was normal, and his hearing problem was due to middle ear infection that it was felt would improve with age.

At preschool, Sam was very sociable. He made friends easily and friends were very important to him. He was full of fun and tended to play rather than paint or draw. His lack of concentration was beginning to be noticed at home. He would only ever sit through half a book or television program. He would sing all the time. Meal times were a very long process of trying to get him to go back to eating his dinner. He was an extremely active little boy from the moment he awoke to the time of going to bed. Sam at this age would go off with anyone. In the park, if another family's picnic looked better than ours he would be off sitting with them instead of us!

At kindergarten, the teachers picked up on the fact that Sam lacked concentration and listening skills. The teacher would ask all the children to get up off the mat and go and do something and Sam would always be sat there wondering where everyone was going. He would hum a lot during class and be totally distracted. He had a very short memory and was never able to complete tasks in the afternoon that he had started in the morning. There was an occasion when Sam was found wandering around the school appearing lost. He had gone to the bathroom and taken a wrong turn and ended up in the school office. This was quite worrying as the school only has three classrooms.

In the second year of school, Sam was selected to have extra help with volunteer readers. This involved one-on-one reading and writing sessions twice a week for half an hour. By the third year of kindergarten, Sam was also having one-on-one daily precision teaching and extra help with the classroom assistant, as well as continued volunteer sessions. Sam's hearing seemed to deteriorate during this time and he was again referred to an ENT consultant. The middle ear infection was bad and it was suggested that if still bad in three months that he have tubes.

The teacher arranged for Sam to see an educational psychologist. After seeing Sam for five minutes she agreed that he needed a full review. Eight months on we are still waiting for this to happen.

Kindergarten was a hard time for Sam. He enjoyed school but found much of it boring as he had no idea what was going on. He went through a period of getting "sad" faces nearly every day so that in the end I started to say well done for only getting one sad face. After pointing this out to the teacher, she agreed that this was not right and that he was not a naughty child and should not be receiving sad faces for being distracted and messing about. This was a very frustrating time for Pete and me. We were concerned that he was not getting enough help in the classroom and worried about how he would cope with going up to primary school.

It was toward the end of his time at kindergarten that we heard about Tinsley House Clinic. Someone who knew of Dr. Pauc's work with children recommended him to us. After an initial consultation, he felt he could help Sam by brain stimulation exercises, a change of diet, and omega-3 and omega-6 supplements. We have now been seeing Dr. Pauc for four months and the difference with Sam is unbelievable. He has started primary school, who say they cannot believe he is the same boy that the teachers wrote about in the kindergarten final assessment. He is so much more confident and able to take part in school activities. His concentration, reading, and writing have improved enormously. His new teacher has mentioned how well he is doing and that she has no issues in the class with him. At home he is much more confident. He can now hold a good conversation and is much more interested in everything. He loves going to see Dr. Pauc because he knows it is helping him at school. His middle ear infection has now gone and he has been discharged from the ENT clinic without any surgery. Things are really looking up for Sam and we thank Dr. Pauc for all his help in achieving this.

AT and PT

Bed-wetting—Simon, aged eleven

*Simon's mother brought him to the clinic without fully realizing what the clinic specialized in. She had heard that the five-year-old son of a friend's neighbor had been cured of his bed-wetting and wondered if I could do the same for eleven-year-old Simon. Chatting to Simon while his mother completed the paperwork was really all I needed to know as to why, at eleven, he still **wet the bed** every night. It was an effort for him to construct and get his sentences out, he **blinked constantly** and had a **minor facial tic**.*

I questioned his mother as to whether there was any family history of learning or behavioral problems. She denied any problems on her side but explained that her ex-husband, Simon's father, had apparently been a "difficult child," was obsessive, couldn't keep still, was constantly on edge, was hypercritical of her and Simon, and prior to the divorce had almost driven her crazy with his increasing paranoid delusions.

*Simon had been born by elective caesarean—a choice heavily influenced by his father—and from day one had failed to thrive. He had suffered from colic, was **late attaining all his developmental milestones**, was struggling at school even though he was considered a bright child, and had gone downhill since the separation and subsequent divorce. He had been treated for asthma, suffered from recurrent bouts of tummy aches, resulting in a lot of time off school, and was prone to frequent headaches.*

Simon's diet consisted of nothing but carbohydrates and water. He did not take part in sport of any kind and his only pastime was computer games. Since the divorce his father had moved abroad but would contact him virtually daily by e-mail telling him how he must work harder at school and excel.

Putting together the information from the consultation and the results of the examination, it became all too obvious that Simon was suffering from a developmental delay syndrome which included symptoms of obsessive-compulsive disorder, Tourette's, minor ADHD, dyspraxia, with secondary ADD and dyslexia—because he couldn't concentrate and learn because of the other symptoms—thrown in for good measure. The bed-wetting was merely a by-product of an under-functioning brain, not helped by the stress generated by the separation, the divorce, and his father's daily e-mails.

Clearly this was not going to be a one-treatment fix, as can happen with younger children, and would require the cooperation of both Simon and his mother. Simon needed help and he knew it, and therefore agreed to a graduated change in his diet. First, no more cereals and toast for breakfast and, once a cooked breakfast was in place, no more pasta for supper. Each week he had to try two new vegetables or fruits and insure by the end of a month he was eating a balanced diet. This was to be supplemented for three months with daily vitamins and a double dose of omega-3 and omega-6.

An exercise regime was put in place that contained specific cerebellar exercises and regular evening walks and talks with his mother. The excessive use of computer games was restricted and replaced by family games he could play with his mother and joining a local judo club.

The tricky bit was to stop the constant criticism he received from his father, or at least get Simon to cope with it better. As it happened, one phone call from Simon's mother somehow did the trick; the e-mails were less frequent and only contained fatherly chat.

Six weeks later the bed-wetting was down to the odd accident, the tic had disappeared and Simon laughed when the odd compulsion came into his mind. The treatment continued over the next few months but I was now treating a happy, confident boy, not a very anxious, frightened child.

The "autistic" label—Chloe, aged seven

Chloe was brought to see me by her mother, despite a very long and difficult telephone conversation, in which I was trying to dodge the issue and not to say, because of the autistic label her mother repeatedly mentioned, "I won't treat your daughter." It was long because her mother wouldn't let me dodge it.

*When Chloe entered the room she appeared to be oblivious of me. She settled on the floor and, in a language I could not comprehend, told her mother what she wanted, which was a bag containing endless pictures which she cut out with great skill using her own scissors. There was no **eye contact** at any point and when I spoke directly to her there was either **no response** or she would say "Ner."*

*Chloe had been **born prematurely** and had spent the first few weeks of her life in the premature baby unit of the local hospital. However, once at home she had achieved all her milestones pretty well on time, taking into consideration her premature arrival, and in* *many ways was an ideal child. This all changed when, following a high temperature round about the time of her MMR, she started to go downhill fast. She **withdrew into herself** and what language she had rapidly disappeared.*

By the time of this consultation Chloe had been everywhere and seen everybody, but to no avail. Having talked things through with her mother I decided I would attempt to examine Chloe over the course of a few visits when I could try to incorporate the tests I needed to do into playful interactions with Chloe—if she would let me. In the meantime I would change her diet, taking out everything that was potentially damaging to her frail developing nervous system and add the essential omega-3 and omega-6.

Judging only by experience and observation I also instituted a series of exercises to be carried out at home on a daily basis, designed to activate the left cerebellum. If Chloe was truly autistic then the chances were that at least some of the brain cells—the spindle cells—that should be produced round about four months after birth would be absent. However, my judgement was that because she had developed normally until the day of the high temperature, sufficient brain cells would be in place for this not to be the case.

After the third visit the bag of pictures and the endless cutting out stopped, we had regular eye contact, we worked on the computer together and, the greatest triumph of all, Chloe shared a piece of her food with me. We have a long way to go, but already after just six visits, she is having to rely less upon signing to fill the gaps in her spoken language, she is behaving more and more like a seven-year-old girl, and I am confident that within a relatively short space of time we will see that miracle her mother so desperately desires.

Now every time I see Chloe I am reminded of her mother's determination to get the right treatment for her child and so very grateful that I did not stick to my original thought not to see her.

Now that we've considered some of the most commonly asked questions and got an idea of what treatment may involve, let's move on to the assessment and the examination.

7

THE ASSESSMENT

If you think that your child may have a learning or behavioral problem you will probably have been to see your doctor and eventually arrived at the point of being ready to have your child assessed by a specialist of some sort. You may have noticed symptoms yourself or have had them pointed out to you by your child's teacher or a family member.

The purpose of this chapter is to help you prepare before the assessment so that you can get the best possible assessment for your child. This will, in turn, help the examination process (which comes after the assessment) to be as accurate as possible, as the examination largely focuses on the picture, or the areas of concern, that were noticed in the assessment.

This chapter will also give you and your child a clearer idea of what to expect in the assessment and what to mention to the practitioner. It will help you to figure out what to ask them if you feel that all bases are not being covered.

Dyslexia?—John, aged eight

Eight-year-old John came to see me with his mother and grandmother. Recently his schoolwork had been going downhill to the point that the school had contacted his parents and arranged a meeting. Previously he had coped at school but now for some reason he was failing to keep up with his peers. He had not been formally tested but now both the school and his parents were concerned that he might be dyslexic.

There was no family history of learning or behavioral problems, he was born at full-term and, apart from needing a little assistance to enter the world, was a healthy baby. He had attained all the developmental milestones on time apart from being a little late gaining bladder control at night. Only on direct questioning did his mother admit that he had always been **a bit clumsy**, putting this down to his being a boy and always on the go.

The medical history was unremarkable apart from some **early eczema** and **recurrent ear infections**. On examination the pieces began to fit together. When tested with a standard eye test he **failed to get halfway up the chart**. Put simply, he would be unable to read anything off the board at school. When tested to see if he could follow an object as it moved toward his nose, his left eye refused to move in. Therefore, not only could he not read what the teacher had written on the board, but he could only look at the book in front of him using his right eye. As he had never suffered from double vision, the information entering his left eye was being "turned off" by the brain. Also, as the eyes are meant to travel across the page together when reading (and this of course was not possible), the right eye would struggle to hold still on a single word or to track across the page. No wonder John was having problems.

His left cerebellar hemisphere was grossly under-functioning, explaining his history of accidents and the lack of left-eye control.

I sent John home with a series of simple exercises to carry out each day to stimulate the left cerebellar hemisphere and a computer-generated program to correct the left-eye problem. I planned on reassessing John in a month using a series of computer-generated tests.

When next we met John was wearing glasses. He had been doing the exercises I gave him, but his mother had obviously decided that a second opinion was also called for and had taken him off to the local optician for an eye test. I asked her if they had done the test to see if the eyes moved in toward the nose. No, they had not. I retested John using the same eye chart without him wearing his glasses. He could now get two-thirds of the way up the chart without a problem.

Four months on and John had near-normal eye control, 20/20 vision and no glasses. He has got a little bit of catching up to do at school but with his newly found perfect vision he should have no problem with that.

THE CONSULTATION

Once you find yourself in a doctor's office you may find that the unfamiliar setting unsettles you as well as your child. You may be worried about what is going to happen next or be so preoccupied with getting your child to behave that you forget the things you want to ask. It is definitely worth thinking about and making a list of the things that you would like to ask before you take your child to be assessed.

You will be asked questions about family history, the pregnancy and the birth of your child, and his or her medical history. All of these questions, answered accurately, will be an enormous help to the accuracy of the assessment and the effectiveness of the treatment.

Before the consultation it might also be helpful to make a list of everything you can remember about your child, no matter how trivial, so that nothing is missed. With the history of the pregnancy and birth, it may help to jot down a brief "story" about how it all went, just to help you to think back to your child's birth and infancy.

Then there will be questions about your child's infancy. Perhaps your child's medical record may jolt some memories of how he or she was as an infant. Family history can be even harder to remember; you may not even have met some members of your family. Ask your parents, aunts and uncles for whatever they can remember about family members.

Dyslexia—Jordan, aged twelve

*Jordan, a twelve-year-old boy, was brought to see me with a classic history of **dyslexia**. Along with the classic history came the typical bundle of documentation including the inevitable psychological assessment. Although such assessments are valuable and provide much detail as to childhood development, they do not in themselves provide an understanding of the underlying problems and therefore of treatment modalities that are desperately needed.*

*The report on Jordan included the comments that he **did not crawl**, was slightly **myopic**, had **poor concentration**, was often **moody**, **anxious**, had **poor personal hygiene** and would respond aggressively by biting when frustrated.*

Reading and writing were major problems, putting him way behind his peers. He was unable to verbalize his needs, gave indications *of having a very **low level of self-esteem** and when **falling over,** as he frequently did, could not tolerate his classmates laughing at him.*

*Along with so many other children, Jordan had suffered from **eczema** most of his life and was prone to **catching anything going around**.*

*On examination Jordan **failed the standard hearing tests,** sat or stood with his **head tilted** to the left, was totally **dyspraxic,** had a marked weakness of the right little finger in abduction—when moving it away from the midline in spreading his fingers—and had a retained primitive reflex indicating that the brain on the right was under-functioning.*

*Although Jordan had arrived already diagnosed as dyslexic, it was apparent from the start that he was also **dyspraxic,** had signs of **attention deficit** and had a few **obsessive-compulsive traits**.*

Jordan was sent home with a set of exercises to perform specifically designed to meet his unique needs. Two weeks later he was seen again, reassessed and treated at the clinic. He was sent home this time with a computer program, designed in Holland, that can be modified to meet the individual needs of the patient. In this particular case Jordan had to use the program daily for two six-minute sessions.

After two weeks the clumsiness had gone, his confidence was rocketing and his schoolteachers had reported back to his parents the remarkable changes they had noticed in him. The teachers were unaware at that time that he was undergoing treatment but they certainly noticed, and appreciated, the results.

Family history

At the start of the consultation the first question to be asked will concern any family history of similar conditions. This is often a difficult question to answer with certainty as the use of terms such as dyslexia and dyspraxia is relatively recent and so older relatives will not have been officially diagnosed; probably your grandad would have been dismissed as just slow or lazy.

Instead you'll have to rely on anecdotal evidence such as family stories or myths. What did they say about Grandad? What sort of person was he? Often the only clues will be comments like "He couldn't write" or "He couldn't read much" or "He was just a bit odd."

For the practitioner this is an important information-gathering opportunity and a chance for us to expand our knowledge in the field of genetics and developmental delay. The more information you can give at this stage the better, as this will not only help with your child's assessment but future research as well.

We stated earlier that it is a genetic probability, not a certainty, that the gene in the parents will cause a problem. Family history gives a lot of clues as to what the problem might be. The father's family history is *particularly* important, and I will put a lot of energy into questioning that branch of the family if time is short.

Tics and Tourette's—Tracy, aged nine

Initially this case history does not sound as if it should be included in this book, but on closer examination it becomes very clear that Tracy had far more wrong with her than would meet the eye. You'll see from this case just how crucial it is to get the right assessment for your child.

Tracy had developed neck pain some two months prior to being seen at the clinic. Her mother was toying with the idea of taking her to a chiropractor, when a family friend suggested that in view of her developmental history it might be better for her to be seen at a specialist clinic.

*Tracy had been born at full-term but had swallowed meconium and required **special care** for a few days in an incubator. (Meconium is the dark-green intestinal contents formed before birth and present in a newborn child.) Meconium aspiration syndrome (MAS), which Tracy had, is an intense inflammatory reaction and airway obstruction resulting in possible respiratory distress of the newborn; it was caused by Tracy breathing in meconium-stained amniotic fluid during her time in the womb or during her birth.*

*Following this initial setback Tracy met all her developmental milestones **apart from crawling**. At three years of age her stools became very loose and for a time there were episodes of fecal soiling. However, since that time she has experienced constipation, requiring daily doses of laxative.*

*Tracy's medical history included **asthma; eczema; recurrent ear infections** resulting in tubes being fitted; an **allergy to blue food colorings;** and right-sided **low-back pain** that radiated to the right leg.*

Although both Tracy and her mother were mainly concerned about her neck pain, it became evident during the consultation and exami-

*nation that the pain Tracy was experiencing was **secondary to a cervical dystonia** (aka a wryneck—a condition where the neck gets locked into position due to the wrong messages being sent to the muscles of the neck on one side). On direct questioning Tracy admitted that she had a compulsion to turn her head to the side, which she did repeatedly; more worryingly, at times she was unaware that she was doing it.*

The greatest difficulty in this particular case was explaining that although the neck pain was, of course, very distressing, it was the dystonia that was the main concern, and focus of treatment. Fortunately, following a short course of treatment at the clinic, together with specific exercises carried out at home, the dystonia abated. The underlying problems that allowed the dystonia to come to the fore were also addressed by therapy carried out at home with just the occasional phone call to monitor progress.

Pregnancy, labor and infancy

The next area of interest will be the pregnancy and several questions will need to be answered about the health and well-being of mother and baby during pregnancy; the level of trauma or intervention during birth; and the health of the child during infancy.

Expect these questions to be asked:

- As far as is known, were the mother and baby well during the pregnancy?
- Were there any health or emotional problems during the pregnancy that could have stressed the mother?
- Did the pregnancy go to full-term of forty weeks?

As I have explained in Chapter 4 all human babies are born prematurely, so if the conventional full-term of nine months is not achieved and the baby is premature in that sense of the word, then there is an extra burden on the developing nervous system. The nervous system will be far less developed than it should be, and often it is down to the skills of the neonatal intensive care unit to insure survival, let alone normal development.

Labor and delivery

Next we need to consider the labor and delivery. We are not entirely sure of what the causal effects of prolonged labor, assisted births and fetal distress have on triggering developmental delay syndrome, but at Tinsley House Clinic we've observed that a large number of children coming for assessment have experienced some type of birth intervention—forceps or ventouse—or the baby suffered fetal distress as reported by the mother.

Fetal distress and how it is detected and reported has changed over the years and far closer monitoring takes place these days. However, a great number of mothers may not have been told directly that their child was suffering, but picked up on odd things being said in the delivery room or by a sudden urgency in bringing in other members of the team.

Our knowledge of the effects of prolonged labor, assisted births and fetal distress as factors in triggering delay syndromes is sketchy and we need to gather as much data as possible. Therefore, anything you can tell the doctor at this point about scans you had, medication you took etc. will help to build a picture of your child's development and may help researchers in the future to discover more about what really happens in the developmental process.

At Tinsley House Clinic we have seen a high number of children with developmental delay syndromes who had assisted births and/or fetal distress. We need to do further work to relate the figures on birth-intervention and fetal distress to the various presentations of developmental delay syndromes to see if there is a common denominator. This is important ongoing research and I hope to be able to provide further updates on my website as they happen.

> *At Tinsley House Clinic we have seen a high number of children with developmental delay syndromes who had assisted births and/or fetal distress.*

Once we have discussed your child's delivery we need to answer the following questions:

- Was the child breast-fed and, if not, why not?
- Did the child vomit, have colic or have problems taking the nipple?
- If the child was bottle-fed, was this because of an inability to suckle or the mother's preferred choice?

These questions are important because breast-feeding is best—it contains all the right ingredients, comes at the right temperature, contains antibodies and comes in an attractive container for a young child. Problems taking the nipple may give a clue of problems with suckling, which itself may provide a clue that something is wrong with either the mouth or throat, or the nerves that control them.

Developmental milestones

Next there will be questions about the developmental milestones.

Important note: all children will differ in their development, some will be faster, some slower, so this should simply be regarded as a guide for the "average" child, and nothing more. There is no need to worry if you find that for any reason your child's behavior does not conform to any of these stages. This is not intended to be a set of hard and fast rules, but merely as broad indications of what you might expect to find.

When did the baby first sit unaided? Generally speaking, sitting unaided may well occur by the sixth month and a delay here may be significant.

Did the baby crawl or was he/she a bottom shuffler? Crawling is thought to be essential for the development of cross-cord reflexes. That is, it is thought that, in part of the spinal cord, what are called interneurons link up in such a fashion that they can generate the complex movements involving both sides of the body. Movements such as walking and swimming rely on these interneurons, which form what are called central pattern generators. A nucleus in the brain stem sends pulses to these central pattern generators that create, once learned, these unconscious movements. Unconscious, because once initiated you don't have to think about walking, etc., it just happens and continues until you want to stop or you trip or slip.

Walking is the next aspect of development that needs to be considered. It may be achieved by the first year but is often delayed in association with other milestones. Clumsiness and falling over or an inability to run smoothly are considered later during the consultation.

The development of speech is a very important area of consideration. Normally we would expect a child within the first year to have a collection of single words that are understandable by those other than the parents or siblings. During the second year two words may be strung together, followed by mini-sentences in year three.

A delay in the onset of speech is often detected early on and referrals for specialist evaluation are usual. However, in terms of dysarthria—difficulty talking—it is not uncommon for a tongue-tied child to be missed. I often ask children to stick their tongues out at me. If the child can protrude the tongue then the frenulum (have a look under your tongue for this) is OK. They seem to enjoy it, and this gives me an opportunity to rule out this not unusual problem.

Bladder control is usually attained by two and a half years by day and a little later at night. A delay in gaining continence gives a good indication as to the state of maturation of the nervous system. Often accidents will occur by day during moments of great excitement and at night when the child is overtired or stressed in some other way.

When was a problem first noticed, and by whom?

This is the next key question. Having gone through the milestones of development it is important to gain some insight into when problems were first noticed and by whom. Was it the mother who first thought there might be a problem, a member of the health team or a teacher? This is important, as teachers pick up educational issues while health professionals pick up medical things and parents pick up on general behavior.

In a recent study at my clinic it was found that the diagnosis was made in the following proportions: by the parents (24 percent), the school (21), a pediatrician (21), a psychologist (18), at a hospital (12), by the family doctor (3) and by a neurologist (1). Although it is perfectly understandable that parents and teachers should pick up on the problem initially, it is of some concern that what is basically a neurological problem only involved a single neurological diagnosis. This has to change if we're to see learning disabilities permanently treated. We simply have got to get the right people looking at this. It is a neurological problem, so we need a neurologist to look at and treat the problem.

Extent and nature of the problem

It is then appropriate to question further, to ascertain the extent and nature of the problem, as it is essential to realize the full extent of the developmental delay. The mistake that is so often made is that the family doctor will latch on to a particular symptom and only consider that aspect of the clinical picture. As this gives an incomplete picture it is not surprising that often the treatments provided are ineffective.

At Tinsley House Clinic we question parents directly to find out about signs and symptoms that might give clues as to what is wrong with the child. Often parents are not fully aware of symptoms unless we make it clear what we are looking for by asking directly. For instance, when the doctor asks about involuntary movements it is important to understand that Tourette's syndrome may show itself as just a repeated clearing of the throat and not necessarily—as many of us may think—a violent tic associated with the odd swear word.

You may have already been given some indication as to what might be wrong with your child. For instance, you may have been told that your child is dyslexic and so you have become quite an expert in looking out for and noting signs of dyslexia, to the exclusion of other symptoms.

Therefore, the consulting physician must ignore any assumptions made and explore every possible avenue and look for other symptoms and signs that will help to build an accurate and complete clinical picture of what is wrong with your child.

To add to the confusion of diagnosing a child, what can also happen is that the parents may think they know what the problem is, but they're focusing on the wrong thing. Let's imagine parents called Bob and Joan, who believe that their son Angus's main problem is bed-wetting (perhaps because it causes disruption to the household in the middle of the night) and that his poor attention is less of a problem. When Angus is examined it may become apparent that ADD is the main problem. Let's look at a real case similar to that of Angus to illustrate my point that sometimes the parent's perception of the child's condition is often formed by what their main concern is and not the reality of the situation.

The bed-wetter—William, aged seven

*Seven-year-old William was brought to see me by his very stressed-out parents concerning his nightly **bed-wetting**. Once seated, his parents* talked at me nonstop concerning the nightly event, their disturbed sleep, their tiredness, the extra washing they had to do. It was all about them, ad infinitum. All the while William sat beside me wriggling on his seat with his head bowed.

At this point I stopped the monologue, and addressed William directly, putting him at ease and letting him know in a roundabout way that I found his parents difficult to deal with. Having regained control I then directed the dialog with the parents in the direction I wanted, away from the cold wet sheets that so disturbed them.

William had been delivered by a **ventouse-assisted birth** and had suffered **fetal distress**. He had been slightly delayed in sitting unaided, **did not crawl** and had **not walked until fourteen months** old. His **speech had been slightly delayed** and he had **not been dry by day until he was four** years old, and had had several accidents since; interestingly, these occurred when he was stressed by school reports and general feedback.

When he was younger he had been **obsessional** about his room and his toys—everything having to be in exactly the right place—and now was like that about his schoolwork. I asked his parents how long he had had the **facial tic**, to which they answered, "What facial tic?"

William was doing all right at school but, although he worked hard, was not achieving the results his parents expected. I asked William if he was happy at school and eventually managed to drag out of him that he found the work hard and was frequently teased by his peers over his clumsiness.

It takes but a few seconds to wet the bed but all day to live with the symptoms of the developmental delay. His very busy middle-management parents focused on the bed-wetting as this directly impacted upon their highly structured existences. They were completely oblivious to the suffering William endured on a daily basis, only made worse by their anger over the wet beds and the consequent belittling treatment of him.

Treating William was the easy part, but getting his parents to see what they were doing to him took a while longer. In this type of situation I often ask the parent/s to come and see me alone so that we can talk through the situation. As diplomatically as possible I can point out how things might have been handled differently, thus de-stressing the responses and providing a more positive attitude that will encourage the child and not dampen their spirits still further.

Further clues may come from parents themselves. Often parents are surprised to realize how childhood problems can be carried over into adulthood. A prime example of this would be obsessional traits presenting in the adult as a degree of orderliness that is viewed as fairly "acceptable," but in fact is bordering on unnatural. We all know someone who clears up behind you with almost military precision and alignment.

During the consultation process I specifically ask questions that will show evidence of symptoms.

- How is the child doing at school? What do the teachers say about him/her?
- Were they or are they clumsy?
- Did they go through a stage when they were obsessed about something or did they have rituals?
- Have they had involuntary movements—grimacing, excessive blinking?
- Are they ever hyperactive?
- Are they forgetful?

It is essential to look at the bigger picture and to delve into aspects of the child's behavior that might give further clues as to the exact nature of their developmental delay. This is essential as the practitioner has at this stage to build a clinical picture and relate any signs and symptoms, as far as possible, to the appropriate areas of the brain and begin to evaluate the effects of any problems present.

THE MATURING OF OUR BRAINS

Remember in Chapter 4 where we said that *all* human babies are born prematurely in the sense that their brain is not complete at birth. They have to be born before the brain is fully mature because otherwise the baby's head would be too big to be born. During the nine months in the womb there wasn't enough time for the very advanced parts of the brain—those parts that make us truly human—to be finished off, so the process has to continue after birth.

What happens is that four months after birth a second wave of very special brain cells—which include the spindle and other cells—develop, move off to where they need to be in the very front of the brain, and hopefully make contact with lots of other brain cells so that this new area of the brain can control all the very special things that we do as humans.

Diaschisis—is a big word for what is said to occur when one area of the brain under-functions and this causes another often distant area of brain to under-function as a consequence.

Think of it as though you were making a car. If the factory up north that supplies the seat for the car that is produced in the south goes on strike, eventually the factory down south grinds to a halt too.

That is also what happens with the brain.

You might know that language is associated generally with the left side of the brain, but there are many other functions that are also located on the right or left side of the brain.

Therefore, subtle clues will guide the physician during the examination process. For instance, a child who prefers a routine, who doesn't like change and is generally nervous may be telling the physician that his two cerebral hemispheres are not in balance and a diaschisis may be present between the side of the brain that is "down" and its opposite cerebellum. If this is the case it would potentially cause an alteration in muscle tone from one side of the body to the other, with noticeable differences between the axial (trunk) muscles and limb muscles.

To a parent's eye, they would see that their child might always have his head tipped to the left, or carry the right shoulder forward with the right arm slightly bent.

Some of the clues are subtle, while others are suddenly blatantly obvious once pointed out. When we describe the examination process in Chapter 8 we will look closely at the examination of the eyes. During the assessment it is important to observe the child closely and look for physical signs that may add to the clues. A head tilt or minor squint will direct the practitioner later during the examination process, but at this time it is worth telling the practitioner if you have observed a tilt or squint or poor posture before. If you are not sure, then searching the family photo albums may provide the answer; again, you are looking for anything unusual in the way people stand, lean or hold their body.

Once the basic questioning has been completed, I then ask the child if they have noticed certain things. Routinely children should be asked about headaches, tinnitus, blurred or double vision, problems with swallowing and faintness or vertigo. It is often surprising for parents to discover that their child, unknown to them, suffers constant headaches, cannot see clearly or suffers from tinnitus. As we will discover later, a significant percentage of young children have problems seeing, either in terms of acuity or convergence.

Acuity—the ability to see well

Convergence/accommodation—the ability to keep focused on an object, such as a pen, as it moves closer to the nose. Both eyes must move toward the nose at the same time and speed (see page 14).

PREVIOUS CONSULTATIONS

The next stage of the consultation is concerned with previous consultations, examinations or treatments. Some parents have amassed volumes of reports, which unfortunately usually contain lots of big words that, in terms of identifying the problem and treating it, mean nothing. The other thing that many parents do when they are looking for some insight into their child's condition is to have their child assessed by a clinical psychologist. This course of action will make you several hundred dollars poorer but it will not bring you any closer to understanding the nature of the condition that has afflicted your child and it certainly won't provide a solution or even suggestions as to effective treatment.

MEDICAL HISTORY

Lastly, it is necessary to go through the child's medical history in some detail. This is completed by providing major headings that the parents can respond to.

Has your child experienced any of the following:

- illnesses—anything more than a cough or a cold?
- operations?
- broken bones?
- being knocked out?
- stitches?
- knocks, bangs, falls, crashes etc.?

I finish off by asking if the child has suffered from recurrent infections, asthma or eczema.

If your child has had more than a few minor accidents it may provide a clue concerning dyspraxic tendencies, but recurrent infections, asthma and eczema are so common that they can also be considered as a symptom of developmental delay.

By far the most common problem associated with developmental delay is "middle ear infections," closely followed by asthma and eczema. This should hardly be surprising, as the brain regulates the autoimmune system and if the brain is not working as it should, then minor infections run riot and allergies abound. Even in the absence of a current ear infection, a history of recurrent infections demands a thorough examination and tests should include tympanometry and otoacoustic emission tests (specialist tests of ear function) as middle-ear problems are frequently found following such a history, and the child may be partially deaf as a result.

In Chapter 10, I explain how a wonderful side benefit of the Tinsley House treatment is that the immune system also benefits from the diet and treatment and that the health problems described above are greatly reduced and in some cases disappear altogether.

THE BRAIN

During the consultation process the physician should take the opportunity to "walk through the brain." That is, to ask the parents and the child questions relating to the function of as many parts of the brain as possible. It is standard practice to start with the pre-frontal lobe and work backwards through the frontal lobe, parietal lobe, occipital lobe and temporal lobe (see illustration of the left side of the human brain on p. 37).

All of the knowledge we have about the functions of the brain is used to consider a child we are assessing. As far as possible, we must try to relate the symptoms not only to a recognized area of function but also to its location if known. For instance, we know that the language centers are usually located in the left brain, while the centers for prosody (the lilt of language) are in the right brain. It is the right brain that sets the timing of the gaps between words and also the inflections in speech and without it the voice is flat, monotone and boring.

However, some functional areas we cannot be certain about. The bladder-control area giving executive control could be bilaterally located, but clinical evidence would suggest, particularly in boys, that it is a right-brain function.

The importance of this exercise is as far as possible to locate areas of the central nervous system that are producing symptoms so that the treatment can be directed specifically at those areas. This may sound obvious, but such a lot of what has been written about dyslexia is so divorced from functional neurology as to make it confusing, if not counterproductive.

Once the assessment is complete, the physician should have a very good idea of just what is going on with the child, and the examination that follows is purely to confirm the impression gained in the assessment. However, often the parents and sometimes the physician are surprised by some very basic findings that have been missed previously. As we said earlier, the mistake that is so often made is that the physician will latch on to a particular symptom and only consider that aspect of the clinical picture. As the clinical picture in this situation is incomplete, the treatments provided are ineffective.

At Tinsley House Clinic we avoid making this mistake by looking to see what other symptoms there are to make the picture as complete as possible before the child is examined.

Now let's move on to the examination itself, which follows the assessment.

8

THE EXAMINATION

The examination follows the assessment for good reason. The information that comes out of the assessment should tell the physician which particular tests are needed.

Reports from educational psychologists may bring various aspects of the impact of developmental delay to the fore, but without relating them to brain structure and function they only end up being expensive words. Optometrists can measure accurately many forms of visual impairment and yet, to date, it has not become standard practice to test for accommodation/convergence failure, which is present in so many children with developmental delay.

As we have already seen, in a recent study of who had made the initial diagnosis of children, only 1 percent had been diagnosed by a neurologist. The neurological examination is a logical process, each part designed to test a specific function of the nervous system. When examining a child with suspected developmental delay it is essential to be both patient and methodical. The defects are often subtle and therefore require experience and careful attention to detail both to detect and interpret.

Here we will describe what you should expect to happen during the examination process and concentrate on the interpretation of the more important findings.

Having noted any observations made during the consultation or assessment process, the neurological examination should start with the cranial nerves, then the cerebellum and lastly the peripheral nerves.

The cranial nerves originate in the brain and brain stem and include the nerves that are involved with the special senses of our sense of smell, taste, vision and hearing. All the tests associated with the cranial nerves need to be carried out as they can provide signs, some obvious and some subtle, that things are not what they should be. For instance, when testing the sense of smell it is important to use easily recognized substances, e.g. orange and peppermint, but also something like cassia oil or cinnamon which, although not known to most individuals, does seem familiar. The reasoning behind this is that the principle association area for smell is in the right frontal cortex, an area of brain we are very interested in knowing about in terms of functioning, as this is where the spindle cells develop and therefore where any delay in development affects the child's ability to mature.

It may seem obvious, but the first test for the eyes that needs to be carried out is for eyesight, using a standard chart just like at the opticians. I say obvious, but a high proportion of the children I examine can't see. That is, they cannot complete the test, which means in the classroom they will struggle to see what has been written on the board. It is difficult to keep up with your peers if you simply can't see what the teacher wants you to.

However, there are other tests for the eyes that are equally vital and if done correctly can provide important clues as to what is happening. Of these tests the most important, and strangely enough the one that is most often omitted, is convergence/accommodation testing. We have found that 58 percent of children have problems with this, which effectively means they cannot see adequately close up. Just think how many children have been labeled as "dyslexic," when in fact their problem is that they cannot see.

If a problem with the eyes is suspected then further testing must be performed using specialist tests including a computer-generated program that can measure the degree of failure both objectively and accurately.

Standard hearing tests need to be backed up by more advanced testing, as hearing impairment is a common finding and, even after the recurrent ear infections have long ceased to be a problem, the middle ear can still be suffering the after-effects. To do this we use special apparatus that prints out the results. This is very important as it provides yet another way that we can monitor the child's progress.

Asking the child to say "Ah" and observing the back part of the roof of the mouth can give another important clue as to the functioning of the two sides of the brain. Often it will be noted that the soft palate in this area fails to elevate as it should on the side that the brain is under-functioning.

THE CEREBELLUM—WHERE THE PROBLEM LIES?

Although it is essential to test the cerebellum it must be borne in mind that it is not the seat of learning disorders, but an area of the brain that provides important clues as to what is going wrong and where.

An estimated 97 percent of children with developmental delay will have a problem with their left cerebellar hemisphere—literally the little brain that lives in the back of the skull and is so important that it can be thought of as the computer that drives the brain. Therefore, it is essential to test this area thoroughly. Clues as to its malfunctioning will already have been provided by the case history, but here we must test it to establish which hemisphere is at fault.

The first test to perform is called the Provoked Rhomberg's test. It consists of having the child stand with their feet together, hands by the side and eyes closed. The physician then attempts to make the child lose balance by tapping the child randomly on the upper arms. The test is said to be positive if the child repeatedly falls in one direction—toward the cerebellar hemisphere that is at fault.

The second test is performed to see if something called dysdiadochokinesia is present (the inability to perform rapidly alternating movements such as turning the hands from facing palm up to facing palm down rapidly while the arms are outstretched). The limb that fails will be on the side of the cerebellum that is failing.

The third test simply involves touching the tip of the nose with the tip of a finger using alternating hands with the eyes closed. Missing the nose or having a minor tremor just before making contact is a positive sign for me that something is wrong—and again the finger that misses the nose will be on the side of the cerebellar hemisphere that is not working as well as it should.

During the cerebellar testing the physician looks for signs that might constitute what in neurology is called dyspraxia. That is, a loss

The Provoked Rhomberg's Test

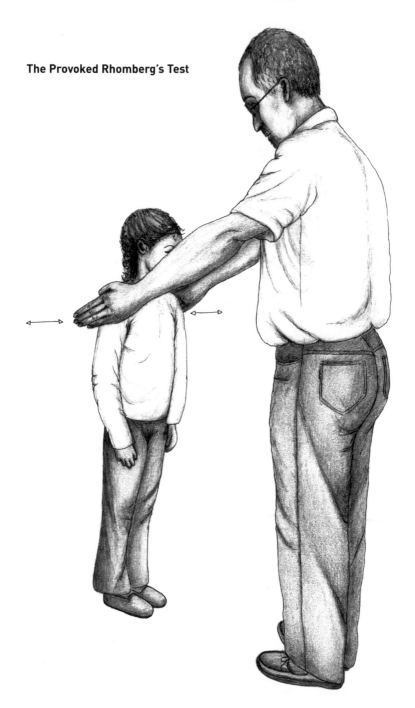

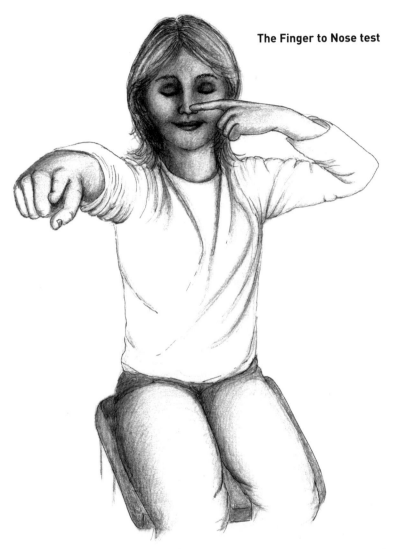

The Finger to Nose test

of coordination of movement or the inability to perform a learned movement.

THE LIMBS

The upper and lower limbs are tested for the ability to sense a light touch, a pinprick and vibration. The muscles are tested for strength and tone and the deep tendon reflexes are tested in turn.

The Babinski sign (the up-going toe test) is looked for when testing the lower limbs. This involves stroking the soles of the feet from the heel up toward the toes and looking to see if the toes spread and/or the big toe goes up. This is a normal sign in infants but should disappear as the brain develops. If still present it represents what is called a retained reflex and is a sign that a cerebral hemisphere is under-functioning (it is not a worrying sign of something else wrong in the central nervous system). If the test is positive, the four corners of the abdomen must be stroked with a sharpish object. The normal response is for the bellybutton to move toward the stimulus.

The assessment should also include discussion of the parent's questionnaires, testing all the cranial nerves—for vision, hearing, etc.—and the cerebellum and peripheral nervous system. How the various signs and symptoms are put together is beyond the scope of this book, but is covered in various papers etc. that can be found on my website (www.tinsleyhouseclinic.com).

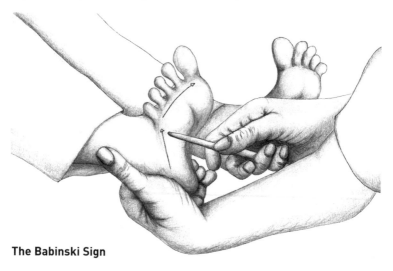

The Babinski Sign

9

FOOD—THE GOOD AND THE BAD

The right food is absolutely vital in helping your child's brain to perform properly. Good foods will support the brain, helping it to develop as it should. Bad foods will harm it and stop it from doing its job properly. That is why, at Tinsley House Clinic, the starting point for treatment for all children with learning and behavioral difficulties is to alter your child's diet to exclude harmful foods and replace them with beneficial foods.

FIVE STEPS TO GET YOUR CHILD'S BRAIN WORKING

The Diet and Supplement Treatment Plan includes the following five steps:

1. reducing food additives in general, and specifically according to the diagnosis;
2. taking out—as far as is humanly possible—artificial sweeteners;
3. reducing carbohydrates;
4. adding omega-3 and omega-6 together with zinc sulfate at the appropriate dosage (see later in this chapter for more information on omega-3 and omega-6);
5. introducing foods that will help the child's brain to function at its best.

Now I'll explain why you should alter your child's diet if they have a learning or behavioral problem.

ARE WE POISONING OUR CHILDREN?

The way we eat and what we eat has changed dramatically over the past few decades. Traditionally, mother would put a meal on the table and that was what the entire family ate. The food would have been bought fresh locally and would be prepared by her, probably using recipes passed down from her mother. This collection of recipes in the UK would include roast dinners for Sundays and special occasions, stews, casseroles, cold cuts with salads, together with various dishes based on fish and offal. The weekly menu would vary but only be based on what was available according to the season or the family income. Many people kept their own chickens and therefore had a plentiful supply of fresh eggs, while others were able to buy them locally from a known source.

Such a diet would be rich in the essential ingredients such as protein, fat, carbohydrate, vitamins and minerals and would come from known sources, often organic and possibly home grown. Obviously there were times—during the Depression, due to a strike or war—when good food was hard to come by, but generally the diet was more than adequate in terms of providing good quantities of the essential ingredients needed for growing bodies and brains.

By contrast, today you can eat virtually anything you want, when you want, regardless of the season. Also, the weekly menu has changed considerably and exotic dishes from around the world are waiting on the supermarket shelf to tempt your palate. In the UK, liver casserole, steak and kidney pie or beef stew with dumpling no longer feature regularly on the menu and, if they do, as often as not a factory somewhere in the world has mass-produced them. Even our eggs are supplied by "factories."

There is a cost: in order for such a wide range of foods to be available, many foods have to be imported, canned, stabilized, chilled, frozen or doctored using some other method so that they remain looking good and have a long shelf life. We no longer know where our food comes from or what has gone into it.

Unfortunately, the problem does not end here, because in this shift away from home-grown or locally produced products, available in season and generally very fresh, we now have the modern-day Aladdin's Cave, the supermarket. Perhaps a better metaphor would be Pandora's Box—open it at your peril.

HOW KIDS DICTATE THEIR DIET

A further threat to the quality of our child's diet comes from children themselves. It used to be that a child would have to eat what was put in front of them or they would go without. That is no longer the case in most families, and parents will often let the child choose the food as they fear that, if they don't, the child won't eat at all.

In many households what is purchased will be influenced or even dictated by the children. Often the children decide upon the menu, whether by making specific requests or by refusing to eat certain things. The parent will often prepare individual meals for the children based on their own particular fads or fancies.

The danger with this situation, in which the child dictates the diet, is that children will often select a high-carbohydrate diet laden with additives and laced with artificial sweeteners. We all know this isn't healthy, but this is more than just an unhealthy diet, it is actually *poisoning* our children.

The main culprits in "poisoning" our children are excess sugar, excess salt and chemical additives. Once I've explained exactly the effect they have on the brain you'll see that I'm not exaggerating when I say "poison."

If you think it is going to be tough to change your child's diet, you're probably right, but it can be done. And it is worth it. My patients do it and reap the rewards for their children, but if my word is not convincing enough for you, it has even been shown on television to work.

We have seen an increasing awareness and debate about the food our children eat in the new millennium, prompted by a rise in childhood obesity and the rise in diabetes. And then in 2005 came UK TV chef Jamie Oliver's program—*Jamie's School Dinners*. He worked hard to get children to eat healthy, properly cooked food by teaching cafeteria ladies to cook and by radically altering the ingredients in the dinners provided in several London schools. He met tough resistance but eventually won most children over.

Many who saw the show will not forget the chicken nuggets

scene, where Jamie offered children a choice of nuggets or pieces of chicken. As you'd expect, they all chose the nuggets. He asked them to hang on a minute while he showed them what the ingredients of nuggets are by making some—from scratch—in front of them. They saw everything that went into the nuggets and were appalled. He offered the plates of nuggets and chicken pieces again. All hands reached out for the chicken pieces. Jamie Oliver also introduced us to the horror that is a turkey twizzler. The media now seems incapable of mentioning children's food without also mentioning turkey twizzlers, an item of food few adults had ever heard of before but few would want to eat.

The show highlighted the nutritionally deficient food that thousands of children in this country are fed every day. The ensuing outcry and media debate actually got the UK Government thinking about what our children were being fed at school and subsequently it has even proposed changes to be made to school dinners in response.

GOOD FOOD IDEAS

1. Getting your oats—a good breakfast option, they contain vitamin B, iron, zinc and calcium plus carbohydrates and fiber
2. Eggs—a good source of choline, vitamins B and E and zinc
3. Nut butters (if no allergy problems)—a good source of the right sort of fat if no hydrogenated fats are mixed in
4. Live yogurt—good if it has no extra additives
5. Melons—contain vitamin C and betacarotene
6. Broccoli—contains B-vitamins, calcium, potassium and betacarotene
7. Sweet potatoes—a good source of betacarotene and fiber
8. Real orange juice (not concentrate or as a bottled fruit drink)—contains vitamins C and E, potassium and zinc

---

WHAT TO LOOK OUT FOR IN FOODS

Over the past few years we have all become familiar with additives. Some people ignore them, others avoid certain of them, and a few

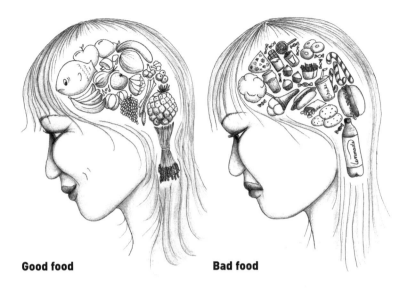

Good food   **Bad food**

people have become self-taught experts. But are they all bad? The answer is certainly not, but in among them are some really bad ones that are banned from human consumption in many nations of the world and yet freely available to consume with abandon in others, including the US.

One would think that if you armed yourself with a list of the worst additives it would be relatively straightforward to check each label of the product before making a purchase. If only that were true. Let us suppose that you have written out your list of additives and headed off for the supermarket to do your weekly shop. However, as you check each product before placing them in your cart, you discover that some of the labels don't have additives as such, but long chemical-sounding words that you can't even pronounce. To buy or not to buy, that is the question. Could it be that the manufacturers have also become concerned about additives and so have effectively removed them from the label but not the product?

Recently I have noticed that certain products no longer contain aspartame. Also, when comparing the label on the front to the label on the back, it is quite easy to get somewhat confused with a lot of products. If the label on the front says "NO ADDED SUGAR" I always ask myself two simple questions: if there is no added sugar, how much was there in the first place. And have they added anything else? Also, have you ever wondered why you can read the words on the front label with ease, while you need a magnifying glass and a good light to read the ingredients listed on the back label?

When looking at the product label, when was the last time you checked the salt content? In fact, do you know the maximum recommended daily intake of salt for an adult and for a child? They are 6g for an adult and 5g for a child aged between seven and ten.

Let us take, for example, a firm favorite with many families, the pan pizza. Obviously the filling will influence the figures, but does 1500 calories, 8.5g of salt and 60g of fat in a pepperoni pizza sound OK? Well, apart from the calories—and there are almost enough here to launch the space shuttle—there is quite a lot of salt and fat. In fact there is 2.5g more salt than the total recommended daily intake for an *adult* male. A recent report by the Foods Standards Agency (UK) found that certain child-size pizzas tested contained 1.4g of salt, while other takeaway pizzas from a well-known outlet contained 2.9g of salt. They also found that a half-can of baked beans from three major supermarkets contained 3.2g of salt. (And beware—the sugar content of your can of beans can vary considerably, often depending on how much you paid for it. The cheaper brands contain more sugar to improve the taste.)

Not to mention all that fat in the pan pizza—if taken on a regular basis it will not only slow down your brain but could well block your digestive system. The constant intake of manufactured foods with a high fat content—burgers, steak pies, bacon and cheese slices, lasagna etc.—does not just lead to a touch of constipation but a complete reversal of the normal digestive process, with that which should exit the body at the bottom having to leave via the mouth. This is a horrifying reality even for some children.

Salt and sugar—everyday evils

We are going to look at all of the evils that can be found in our children's food. Before looking at the additives that have been implicated in generating the symptoms of the developmental delay syndromes, we must first look at other health issues associated with the addition of salt and sugars to food targeted at children.

In a recent report by the UK magazine *Which?* the salt and sugar contents of the top ten breakfast cereals were examined. The results were shocking, revealing far higher amounts of both than listed in the recommended daily intake for children aged between seven and ten.

Imagine, if 49 percent of your child's favorite breakfast cereal is sugar, when the child sprinkles still more sugar on the top it becomes rocket fuel. When considering sugars you have to bear in mind that some sugars are rapidly taken into the bloodstream while others, for instance fructose in fruit, have to be processed within the body and are therefore said to be slow-release sugars. What this means in effect is that some sugars will provide a rapid rise in blood-sugar levels which will equally rapidly fall off, while other sugars will provide a slower release, thereby helping to prevent unhealthy fluctuations.

Perversely, the brain enjoys these sugar highs and this would appear to trigger a specific area of the brain, the pleasure center, which then craves the next high. Hence the all-too-common mood swings seen in children on high-sugar diets.

A spoonful of sugar—why do kids love it so much?

Breast milk contains lactose, a sugar which gives it a slightly sweet taste and might provide the starting point of many children's love of all things sweet. Our tongues have specialized taste buds capable of detecting combinations of the basic tastes—sweet, salty, bitter and sour—but it would seem that there is a particular liking for the sweet taste, perhaps given by Nature to insure that the baby feeds.

This preference for sweet things can become a problem in that children may opt for a high-carbohydrate/sugar diet, which may also include substantial quantities of artificial sweeteners. Before looking at the problems associated with certain foods we must look at the nature of these foods and the different types of sugars and sweeteners that occur in our diets.

Carbohydrates are foods that provide energy to living cells. The carbohydrates we use as foods have their origin in the process of photosynthesis—sunlight falling on chlorophyll in plants. They take the form of sugars, starches and cellulose.

Sugars are those carbohydrates which are used directly to supply energy to living organisms. Table sugar—sucrose—is a disaccharide (glucose/fructose) and provides about 16 calories per teaspoonful. Fruit sugar—fructose—also provides 16 calories per teaspoonful (or 4 calories per gram).

Artificial sweeteners provide the sweet taste desired by many consumers but have no or only a few calories to accompany that taste. Sweeteners can be hundreds or thousands times sweeter than sugars and therefore are only required in tiny amounts to provide the desired effect. In a world dictated by fashion they have become increasingly popular as tabletop sweeteners (the ones we add to food ourselves rather than being added in manufacture) and as part of a calorie-controlled diet—but at what cost?

The top six low-calorie sweeteners are acesulfame potassium, aspartame, neotame, saccharin, sucralose and tagatose.

- **Saccharin** (e.g. Sweet'N Low) is the oldest sugar substitute. It is 300 times as sweet as sugar and is a very popular tabletop sweetener. Since its discovery in 1879 it has had a checkered history, being used during both world wars, helping to compensate for sugar shortages and rationing, and in the 1970s being suspected of causing bladder cancer in laboratory animals. Depending upon which side of the fence you sit, either as manufacturer or consumer, it is either perfectly safe or is a carcinogen.
- **Aspartame** (e.g. NutraSweet/Equal) has a history that could easily be rewritten as a bestselling thriller. It has been alleged that it can cause a host of conditions including brain tumors, seizures, birth defects, multiple sclerosis and lupus. Headaches and dizziness have been reported following aspartame ingestion but to what extent this occurs within the population is not known. In the context of developmental delay aspartame has been implicated in what has been called "glutamate storms." That is, it would appear that aspartame triggers a cascade effect whereby excessive amounts of glutamate (an excitatory neurotransmitter) are liberated, resulting in hyperactive and often pointless destructive behavior in children. Anyone with any doubts as to whether or not to avoid aspartame only needs to do a little homework on the Internet.

- **Acesulfame potassium** (e.g. Sunett/Sweet One) is often combined with other sweeteners when used as a food additive. It would appear that it has not been tested as thoroughly as some of the other sweeteners, so therefore researchers tend to be less well informed concerning possible side effects.
- **Neotame** is made from the same two amino acids that are used to make aspartame. However, unlike aspartame the chemical bond between the amino acids is stronger and neotame is not broken down in the process of digestion and phenylalanine is not therefore produced.
- **Tagatose** (e.g. Naturlose) is derived from lactose. There has been some debate as to the safety of the method of manufacture and claims for its use in the management of diabetes type II.
- **Sucralose** (e.g. Splenda) is made from sugar in a complex multi-step process. It is 600 times as sweet as sugar, is not digested and does not raise blood-glucose levels. Based on current information, that makes this the best of the bunch at present.

The reason for looking at sugars and artificial sweeteners is the possible impact they have on children with developmental delay syndromes. It would appear that many of these children have a sugar addiction—maybe starting from the sweetness in breast milk—causing them to crave a high-carbohydrate/sugar diet.

During the process of growth and development the nervous system, along with the rest of the body, obviously needs fuel—oxygen and glucose—but it doesn't need too much at any one time. Children who are fussy eaters insidiously create their own diet, often based on nothing but carbohydrates and pure sugars. This floods the system with too much fuel and causes a temporary high, which the brain enjoys, and this triggers a specific area of the brain, the pleasure center, which then craves the next high. Mothers are often duped into providing their children with the foods they want and fuel the cravings by feeding the children with potato chips and high-glucose drinks. It is not unusual for children to have cereal and toast for breakfast, potato chips and cookies mid-morning, pizza and fries for lunch, more potato chips, cookies and cake mid-afternoon, and hamburgers and fries for supper.

Unfortunately, there is a second complication to this child-driven diet in that it often contains high levels of additives and artificial sweeteners. We have already mentioned the possible dangers involved with aspartame usage and this is no more true than in the case of children who have as their prime symptom attention deficit and hyperactivity.

SUGAR ADDICTION: THE BEGINNINGS OF AN ADDICTIVE PERSONALITY?

Earlier we talked about sugar addiction and the likelihood of a child developing an addictive personality. There is evidence that there may be a genetic basis to addiction, but the expression of that gene or genes may result from something as simple as giving the brain too much sugar while it is immature and still developing. That is, we know that it is perfectly possible for a person to carry a gene for a particular disorder without that disorder occurring. However, it would appear that certain things can act as triggers and cause the gene that has been lying dormant to wake up, and the disorder then starts to appear.

It may well be that tickling the brain's pleasure center is all that it takes to set off a chain of events that can lead to a lifetime of addiction, whether it is smoking, alcohol or so-called recreational drugs. All will have an impact on the lifestyle, health and finances of your child.

Nearly every child treated at Tinsley House Clinic is put on a low-carbohydrate, high-protein (to build the body), good-fat (to build the brain) diet for two weeks. What we aim to achieve with this diet is the avoidance of anything that will potentially upset the brain. It is of interest to note that recent research in the USA has found that patients suffering from epilepsy, that did not respond to drug therapy, responded favorably to low-carbohydrate, high-protein, good-fat diets.

In addition, as far as possible, additives are eliminated from the diet along with artificial sweeteners. Generally speaking this makes a significant difference in children whose primary symptom is hyperactivity. After two weeks the diet is modified slightly allowing a little more carbohydrate consumption, but this must be closely monitored.

Additives and behavior

Sugars will be absorbed and in the bloodstream within minutes. Therefore the effects can be pretty well instant and last for a variable period depending on the dose. Bad additives can take a little longer to be absorbed so the effects may not be so instant but when they kick in, they can wreak havoc!

Another aspect highlighted in the UK TV program *Jamie's School Dinners* was the link between diet and behavior. There was a clear improvement in the behavior of the children who had switched to healthier school dinners: they were calmer and concentrated better in class. This is because additives cause hyperactivity and a healthier diet helps the children to be more even-tempered.

The scientific proof

For anyone in doubt as to whether or not additives cause hyperactivity, there is more substantial evidence from a study carried out by Professor John Warner at Southampton University, UK.

This study assessed 277 children over a period of four weeks for levels of hyperactivity. In the first week they were all given a normal diet (that is, everyday foods that may or may not contain additives) followed in the succeeding weeks by an additive-free diet, a diet containing colorings and preservatives, and lastly a diet containing dummy—placebo—additives.

The findings

The parents of these children noticed a distinct rise in levels of hyperactivity during the period when the children were being provided with additives and a lowering of these levels when the additives were withdrawn.

The additives that were used in this trial were tartrazine, sunset yellow, carmoisine, ponceau 4R and sodium benzoate. What is truly amazing about this trial is that the total quantity of additives used was only 5mg per day, while it is estimated that the average child consumes in the region of 20mg a day.

What you need to know about additives

The supermarket shelves and chiller cabinets are stacked with foods to tempt the appetite, but do they contain more than meets the eye? What exactly is an additive?

Additives, as the name would imply, are various substances added to food to preserve it, color it, flavor it, control it, stabilize it, sweeten it, emulsify it, bleach it or enhance it.

Additives can be placed into various categories depending upon their general function, though some can perform more than one function.

Acidity regulators change or maintain the acidity or quality of the base substance of foods and include buffers, acids, alkalis and neutralizing agents that can alter or control the acidity or alkalinity to provide the desired effect, e.g. tartness or preservation, color retention or co-working with raising agents by releasing carbon dioxide.

Anti-caking agents are physical rather than chemical agents—though still chemicals—and are said to be bland and harmless. They alter the physical properties of food and thereby how it handles. They have become an essential part of the fast-food industry, preventing coagulation and agglomeration.

Anti-foaming agents are incorporated into certain foods to prevent or reduce frothing on boiling and the production of scum.

Antioxidants are used to prevent or slow down the process of oxidation, which is the deterioration of the food on exposure to air, such as color fading, flavor reduction or fat rancidity.

Bleaching agents are used to whiten flour and are often used with flour improvers that accelerate the action of bleaches and themselves enhance the elastic nature of dough and its development.

Bulking agents do exactly as you would expect and simply add bulk to the food, padding out expensive ingredients or providing roughage. Thus they can increase the volume of a food without significantly adding calories.

Carriers are used not to modify the food but to change an additive either by dissolving, diluting or dispersing it. They are therefore sometimes called carrier solvents.

Colorants are added to colorless foods to make them more appealing, to insure uniformity of color or to preserve color during processing or storage.

Emulsifiers aid in the formation of an emulsion, that is, the mixing of two or more substances that would normally separate. The classic example would be oil and water.

Firming agents are used to keep fruit and vegetables crisp and firm.

Flavorings are used to keep, restore and reinforce the flavor or add a flavor. Flavor enhancers are added to enhance the flavor without directly imparting their own distinct flavor. Bear in mind that if the label says "peach flavor" it only means "flavor" and not that the product contains peaches or peach products.

Humectants are hygroscopic (water-attracting) substances that are incorporated in foods to promote the retention of moisture or its attraction from the air.

Modified starches are used to add texture or bulk or to act as stabilizers.

Packaging gases are used to replace the air in sealed packages of foodstuffs, thus preventing oxidation.

Preservatives are a class of additives designed to prevent bacterial growth and potential food poisoning. Various methods have been tried for generations, from salting to modern-day additives.

Propellants are gases or volatile liquids added solely to provide the pressure needed within a sealed container to propel the foodstuff from an aerosol.

Releasing agents are purely used to prevent the foodstuff during processing or packaging from sticking to the machinery. They are not intended to be included in the product but traces may be carried over.

Sequestrants are used to prevent a chemical effect by combining with trace metals found in certain foodstuffs.

Stabilizers are added so that foodstuffs retain their physical state, color and appearance. They are often combined with emulsifiers.

Sugars and sweeteners are added to adjust the taste of foodstuffs. However, in terms of developmental delay they are potentially a major problem and will be addressed again later.

There is the question as to which additives can be added to foods and the quantities permitted. This is controlled by legislation in many countries, so the type and quantity allowed is controlled by law to keep their use within safe limits. Unfortunately, this would not appear to take into account variations in tolerance to these additives, nor the possible side effects of their consumption.

Food additives

We must now further enter the mysterious world of food additives and try and make some sense of what appears to be a baffling array of chemical names designed to confuse even the most careful shopper. To begin to understand this frightening collection of chemical names we will limit our consideration here to the additives that have been implicated as being harmful to babies, hyperactive children, asthmatics and aspirin-sensitive individuals, and those that are possible carcinogens (a substance that may cause cancer).

The Hyperactive Children's Support Group (HCSG) UK has cited the following additives to which, in their opinion, children may react badly. This group of additives contain azo dyes and benzoate preservatives.

Azo dyes are any of a large class of synthetic organic dyes. In terms of additives they are sometimes classed according to their colors.

The yellow family

Quinoline is a colorant produced from synthetic coal tar. It is banned in Norway, Australia, USA and Japan. It is found in smoked fish and ice cream.

Sunset yellow is a colorant produced from synthetic coal tar and an azo dye and banned in both Norway and Finland. It is added to many food products and is found in many children's favorites, including candy, cakes, yogurts, trifles, orange fruit drink and hot chocolate. It is also found in breadcrumbs, so both home-made and prepared fish fingers and chicken nuggets may be suspect.

Tartrazine is a yellow azo dye that can cause symptoms of asthma, migraine or skin irritation. Its use is banned in Austria and Norway. It is commonly found in fruit concentrates and bottled drinks, cordial and colored sodas which may also contain aspartame. Convenience foods, cake mixes, soups, custard powder, instant desserts, preserves, sauces and salad dressings, mustard and pickles may all contain tartrazine, as do many foods targeted at children including jellies, ice cream, lollipops, yogurt and candy.

Yellow 2G is produced from synthetic coal tar and an azo dye. It is currently the subject of a proposed EU ban.

The red family

Amaranth is a purplish-red azo dye and synthetic coal-tar-based colorant. It is banned in Norway and the USA and is limited in its usage in France and Italy. It is found in canned and packet foods including cake and trifle mix, ices, jellies, gravy granules and, worryingly, liquid vitamin-C preparations.

Carmoisine is a red azo dye that may cause allergic reactions. It is commonly found in candy, ice creams, yogurts, cakes and desserts. It is currently banned in Norway, Sweden, USA and Japan.

Cochineal is a red colorant obtained from pregnant scaled insects. The relatively high cost of this colorant has caused it to be replaced by ponceau, another suspect on the HCSG list. As far as children are concerned it may be found in soft drinks, sugar confectionery, cream cookies and desserts.

Erythrosine is a red colorant made from an azo dye and synthetic coal tar, which again is banned in Norway and the USA. Unfortunately, it is found in many foods targeted by children, including trifles, custard, cookies, cakes, chocolates, canned cherries, strawberries and rhubarb.

Ponceau is a brilliant-red colorant made from an azo dye and synthetic coal tar. It has been said that it should be avoided by asthmatics and those people sensitive to aspirin. It is banned in Norway and the USA. Its use is widespread and includes candy, ices, yogurts, cakes, desserts, preserves, brown sauce, convenience foods and breadcrumbs.

Red 2G is widely banned throughout the world. It is found in meat products and drinks.

The blue family

Brilliant blue is a blue coal-tar colorant that can be used in conjunction with tartrazine. It is banned widely in Europe (though not in the UK) and is found in canned processed peas.

Indigo carmine is a blue coal-tar derivative. It is banned in Norway. It is found in candy and cookies as well as savory prepared foods.

The brown and black family

Brilliant black is a black colorant made from an azo dye and synthetic coal tar and is used in blackcurrant cheesecake mix, brown sauce and chocolate mousse. It is banned in Norway, Finland, Japan, Canada and the USA.

Brown FK is a mix of azo dyes and is used in chips and cooked ham. It is banned within the EU (except the UK), Norway, Canada, Japan, Australia and the USA.

Caramel provides a dark-brown coloring and is found in cola, canned sauces and gravy.

Chocolate brown is an azo dye and synthetic coal-tar mix used in chocolate-cake mixes. It is banned in Australia, Austria, Belgium, Denmark, France, Germany, Norway, Sweden, Switzerland and the USA.

Plant extract family

Annatto provides a peach coloring and is obtained from the seeds of the annatto tree. It is found in certain cheeses, instant mash, cooking oils, meatballs, fish fingers, chips, ice cream, lollies, yogurts, custard, cakes and soft drinks.

Benzoate family

Benzoic acid is a preservative used in soft drinks, fruit juices, fruit yogurt and dessert sauces.

Sodium benzoate is another preservative and is found commonly in candy, fruit pies, soft drinks including orange fruit drink and barbecue sauce.

Sulfur dioxide

Sulfur dioxide is one of the oldest preservatives known to man. It is used in fruit salads, fruit juices, fruit-based desserts, fruit-based pie fillings, fruit spreads, soft drinks and sausage meat.

Sodium nitrate/nitrite

Sodium nitrate is a preservative found in bacon, pressed meats, ham, certain cheeses and frozen pizza.

Sodium nitrite is a preservative targeting clostridium botulinum and is used to prevent food poisoning. It is also found in cured meats, pork sausages, bacon, ham and frozen pizza.

Butylated family

Butylated hydroxyanisole is added to retard products from becoming rancid. It is found in convenience foods, candy, cookies, soft drinks, cheese spread and chips. It is banned in Japan.

Butylated hydroxytoluene again retards rancidity in foods. It is found in chips, salted peanuts, gravy granules, dry breakfast cereals and the packaging inside a cereal box, convenience foods and chewing gum.

Babies and young children should not be given:

butylated hydroxytoluene (BHT)
calcium benzoate
calcium diglutamate
disodium 5'-ribonucleotide
disodium guanylate
disodium inosinate
dodecyl gallate
ethyl p-hydroxybenzoate
mannitol
methyl p-hydroxybenzoate
monopotassium glutamate
monosodium glutamate (MSG)
octyl gallate
propyl gallate
propyl p-hydroxybenzoate
sodium ethyl p-hydroxybenzoate
sodium methyl p-hydroxybenzoate
sodium propyl p-hydroxybenzoate
sulfur dioxide

Many children with developmental delay syndromes also suffer from eczema, asthma and recurrent infections, due to their autoimmune system not working properly, so it is suggested that they avoid:

allura red
amaranth
azorubine
brilliant black
brown FK
brown HT

butylated hydroxytoluene (BHT)
calcium benzoate
calcium diglutamate
calcium hydrogen sulfite
calcium sulfite
disodium 5'-ribonucleotide
disodium guanylate
disodium inosinate
dodecyl gallate
ethyl p-hydroxybenzoate
latolrubine BK
mannitol
methyl p-hydroxybenzoate
monopotassium glutamate
monosodium glutamate (MSG)
octyl gallate
ponceau
potassium benzoate
potassium metabisulfite
potassium sulfite
propyl gallate
propyl p-hydroxybenzoate
red 2G
sodium benzoate
sodium ethyl p-hydroxybenzoate
sodium hydrogen sulfite
sodium metabisulfite
sodium methyl p-hydroxybenzoate
sodium propyl p-hydroxybenzoate
sodium sulfite
sulfur dioxide
sunset yellow
tartrazine
yellow 7G

Some additives *may* be carcinogens—cancer causing—and it is suggested that the following be avoided for that reason:

amaranth

butylated hydroxyanisole (BHA)
butylated hydroxytoluene (BHT)
erythrosine
paraffins (microcrystalline wax)
potassium nitrate
potassium nitrite
refined microcrystalline wax
saccharines
sodium nitrate
sodium nitrite
sunset yellow
vegetable carbon

Some additives have been implicated in causing or aggravating problems with the kidneys and these are:

calcium carbonate
calcium disodium EDTA
calcium phosphates
diphosphates
mannitol
polyoxyethylene (8) stearate
polyphosphates
potassium nitrate
potassium phosphates
sodium aluminium phosphate
sodium phosphates

Finally, if you are a vegetarian you should avoid:

cochineal (carminic acid, carmines)
gelatine
edible bone phosphate
L-cysteine
L-cysteine hydrochloride
L-cysteine hydrochloride monohydrate
lactitol

and limit:

acetic acid esters of mono- and diglycerides of fatty acids

ammonium phosphatides
calcium lactate
calcium stearoyl-2-lactylate
canthaxanthin
carotene
citric acid esters of mono- and diglycerides of fatty acids
disodium 5'-ribonucleotide
disodium inosinate
fatty acids salts (magnesium salts of fatty acids)
fatty acids salts (sodium, potassium and calcium salts of fatty
    acids; emulsifier and anti-caking agent)
ferrous lactate
glycerol
glycine
lactic acid
lactic acid esters of mono- and diglycerides of fatty acids
lactylated fatty acid esters of gylcerol and propane-1,2-diol
lecithins
magnesium stearate
mixed acetic and tartaric acid esters of mono- and diglycerides of
    fatty acids
mono- and diglycerides of fatty acids
mono- and diacetyl tartaric acid esters of mono- and diglycerides
    of fatty acids
polyglycerol esters of fatty acids
polyglycerol polyricinoleate
polyoxyethylene (20)
polyoxyethylene (40) stearate
polyoxyethylene (8) stearate
polysorbate 20
polysorbate 40
polysorbate 80
potassium lactate
potassium nitrate
propylene glycol esters of fatty acids
sodium lactate
sodium stearoyl-2-lactylate
sorbitan monolaurate
sorbitan mono-oleate

sorbitan monopalmitate
sorbitan monostearate
sorbitan tristearate
stearic acid
stearyl tartrate
sucroglycerides
sucrose esters of fatty acids
tartaric acid esters of mono- and diglycerides of fatty acids
thermally oxidized soya bean oil interacted with mono- and
    diglycerides of fatty acids
vegetable carbon

So just how do you cope with additives? Either, move to Norway, petition the government or start off avoiding the list of foods that follows and then make your own list of additives from those given above and check all your food shopping. It may appear daunting but in a few weeks you will have become an expert and then you can ask the supermarket manager why he is selling products known to be harmful and banned in many countries.

FOODS TO LOOK AT CLOSELY FOR ADDITIVES:

Cookies, breadcrumbs, brown sauce, cakes, chicken nuggets, cola, convenience foods, potato chips, cured meats, custard, desserts, fish fingers, frozen pizza, fruit products, gravy granules, hot chocolate, ice cream, instant desserts, jellies, lollipops, orange fruit drink, processed peas, soft drinks, candy, canned fruit, trifles, yogurt.

WHAT IS THAT IN MY FOOD?

Avoid these:

Calcium carbonate—found in bread, cookies, cakes and tooth-paste (source—chalk and sea snails)
Cochineal—found in curries and many types of candy (source—crushed carcasses of the female cactus-feeding coccid insect)
Silicon dioxide—found in instant coffee and some brands of hot chocolate (basically sand)
Shellac—a lot of shiny candy is coated in shellac (source—secreted by the female coccus lacca insect)

FOOD ADDITIVES TO AVOID

Based on information from the ministries of health of the United States, France, England and Russia, the following additives are described as:

Artificial sweeteners—aspartame and saccharin
Suspicious—aluminum, azorubine, brilliant black, caramel, carbon black, carmoisine, copper complexes of chlorophylls and chlorophyllins, lithol rubine BK, quinoline, rubine, titanium dioxide, vegetable carbon
Dangerous—carmines, carminic acid, cochineal, erythrosine, ponceau, sunset yellow, tartrazine
Very dangerous— amaranth
Cancerous—benzoic acid, calcium benzoate, ethyl para-hydroxy-benzoate, greens S, hexamethylene tetramine, hexamine, patent blue, potassium benzoate, sodium benzoate, sodium ethyl para-hydroxybenzoate, sodium propyl para-hydroxy-benzoate

RECOMMENDED DAILY INTAKE OF SUGAR

Sugar does not have a recommended dietary allowance as it is not a required nutrient and therefore does not offer a nutritional value.

DAILY NUTRIENTS AND CALORIES

- Fats provide 9 calories per gram.
  Your child's diet should contain no more than 30 percent of calories derived from fat.
- Carbohydrates provide 4 calories per gram.
  In a normal diet 50–60 percent of calories should come from carbohydrates (sugars, starches and fiber). No more than 10 percent of the total calories should be derived from sugar. This equates to about 50g or 10 teaspoons of simple sugars per day.
- Sodas contain 34–52g of sugar per 330ml can.

Don't be put off by the facts and figures—what they mean is that it is essential to reduce junk-food intake.

RECOMMENDED DAILY INTAKE OF SALT

Age	Grams of salt (also labeled as NaCl—sodium chloride)
0–12 months	Less than 1g
1–3 years	2g
4–6 years	3g
7–10 years	5g
11–Adult	6g (I suggest 5g for a female as they generally have less body mass)

At this point let's put what we have said so far into perspective. During the process of development the nervous system needs a balanced diet to provide all the building blocks required for growth; particularly it needs certain fats to provide the insulating material myelin, which will cover the fast-conducting nerve fibers both in the central nervous system (brain and spinal cord) as well as in the peripheral nervous system (nerves that enter and leave the spinal cord and brain stem).

As we've discussed, children who are fussy eaters insidiously create their own diet often based on nothing but carbohydrates and pure sugars. This floods the system with too much fuel, causing a temporary "high" which triggers a craving for the next fix. Parents desperate for their kids to eat may unwittingly provide their child with the foods that fuel the cravings by feeding the child with potato chips and high glucose drinks.

A further complication with this child-driven diet is that it often contains levels of stabilizers, colorants, and other substances with which the immature brain cannot cope.

Aspartame, used in many soft drinks, juices and foods, has been implicated in what have been called "glutamate storms," resulting in hyperactivity and often pointless destructive behavior in children.

Just to qualify the difference, destructive behavior is when you destroy something for a reason—Sally annoys Stephen so he retaliates by breaking her toy. Pointless destruction is when Stephen goes "crazy" and smashes everything in sight.

So if too much fuel and excessive additives are beyond the developing brain's ability to cope with, what can the parent do to help? The Tinsley House Clinic Eating Plan (see Chapter 11) provides recipes (see the section at the back of the book) and detailed menus of what your child should be eating. The following are some general rules for healthy eating to support your child's brain.

SIX GOLDEN RULES FOR A HEALTHY BRAIN

There are six golden rules for your child's diet:

1. Rule out cereals and toast for breakfast every day and introduce egg and bacon or porridge.

2. Cut out all snack foods, e.g. potato chips, chocolate, sodas, and check all other labels carefully for additives.

3. If you are providing a packed lunch avoid the easy way out of providing prepared and snack foods and use a little creativity that just might tickle your child's appetite (see the recipe section for ideas).

4. Introduce more fruit into the diet—this can replace the snack children often have on getting home from school.

5. The evening meal should be home-cooked and contain fresh meat/fish and vegetables—if you are finding it difficult to get your child to eat fruit and vegetables why not use a juice maker and produce your own exotic cocktails or smoothies (see the recipe section for ideas).

6. Carbohydrates should be provided in moderation.

At all cost parents must avoid the scenario in which the child dictates their diet. Every child needs the best diet possible to enable them to properly develop—even a child without DDS would exhibit wobbly behavior on a diet of toast, potato chips, cookies mid-morning, pizza, burgers, fries, cake and pasta. Sadly, it is not an uncommon diet for children today.

THE GOOD NEWS

The good news is that just two weeks on a modified diet may well be enough in itself to bring about a dramatic change in a child's behavior patterns and reduce levels of hyperactivity considerably.

Now I've told you what your child *shouldn't* be eating, and the additives you should be avoiding. Exactly what your child needs to eat will be covered in detail in the Tinsley House Clinic 14-Day Eating Plan in Chapter 11, with some simple recipes that your kids will love at the back of the book.

But before we get to the food plan, I will first explain the benefits of eating well for your child's immune system, and also how food supplements can help.

10

FOOD SUPPLEMENTS AND THE IMMUNE SYSTEM

FOOD SUPPLEMENTS SUPPORT THE BRAIN

It is precisely because most of our food is mass-produced as well as additive-, sugar- and salt-laden that our diets are deficient in terms of certain vital nutrients. This can be easily remedied by supplementing our diets. Getting the right nutrients is particularly essential for a growing child.

> *The exciting news is that supporting the brain with the right food will help your child's brain develop as it should or will help to redress an underdeveloped brain. As an added bonus it will also boost your child's immune system.*

It is widely accepted that it is beneficial to add multivitamins and minerals as a supplement if your child's diet is not as good as it could be. If your child is following a good diet, vitamins may not be necessary, but additional omega-3 can only do good as it is not present in sufficient quantities even in a good diet. Supplementing your child's diet is particularly important if your child is known to have developmental delay syndrome. Supporting the brain with the right food will help your child's brain develop properly and will boost your child's immune system.

FATS YOU NEED

A lot of press coverage has been given to the effectiveness of omega-3 and omega-6 supplements for children. Apart from being good for your eyes, skin, joints, etc., they are *essential* to brain functioning and help with concentration, making children (and adults) more alert and able to cope with day-to-day life as well as their schoolwork.

There is now sufficient research evidence to show that a great many children would benefit from supplementing the essential fatty acids, and further evidence would suggest that supplements may also ward off the fading memory often associated with ageing, if not Alzheimer's itself.

Children identified as having developmental delay syndromes will especially benefit from having omega-3 and omega-6 added to their diet. In fact it is an absolutely essential part of the Tinsley House Clinic Treatment Plan.

Typical signs of deficiency in children include symptoms such as learning disabilities, poor short-term memory, poor concentration, clumsiness, visual disturbances, recurrent infections and allergies. It is not just children who suffer from essential-fat deficiency. Adults can also manifest subtle signs of deficiency that may surprise you—thirst, itchy dry eyes, raised cholesterol, raised blood pressure and inflammatory diseases such as arthritis.

The science

As this is an area of confusion to many people it is perhaps worth while getting just a little technical at this point.

The process of myelination—the covering and insulating—of nerves requires fat. In fact your brain consists of 60 percent fat. So certain fats are not only good for you, they are essential, and no more is this true than in the case of the brain suffering from a developmental delay.

Research has left no doubt that we require fats as part of our daily diet, from development in the womb, right the way through to old age. The question is, which fats? Saturated fats, monounsaturated fat and cholesterol can be produced within the body, but the polyunsaturated fats (omega-3 and omega-6) have to be obtained through our diet or supplements. Together, the saturated and unsaturated fatty acids form the phospholipids that make up the myelin sheath that surrounds the neurons (nerves) and protects it.

The good fats—monounsaturated fat
Found in: avocado, olives, nuts, sesame seeds, peanut butter, olive oil, canola oil, peanut oil and sesame oil

The good fats—polyunsaturated fat
Found in: walnuts, pumpkin seeds, sunflower seeds, corn oil, safflower oil, soybean oil and cottonseed oil

The bad fats (ones to avoid)—trans fat/saturated fat
Saturated fats found in: animal fat, coconut oil, palm oil, palm kernel oil
Trans fats found in: cookies, commercially fried foods

Essential fatty acids include arachidonic, linoleic and linolenic acids. They all act as precursors (forerunners) to prostaglandins. Put simply, prostaglandins are a group of organic compounds derived from essential fatty acids that cause a range of physiological processes to take place. They are essential to the smooth running of your bodily processes and reduced levels have been thought to cause hypertension, ADD, depression and schizophrenia.

Omega-3 is a family of unsaturated essential fatty acids. A key reason why supplementing is necessary is that the omega-3 family is prone to damage during over-cooking and processing. With the omega-3 family—alpha-linolenic acid, eicosapentaenoic acid (EPA) and docosahexaenoic acid (DHA)—there are two things we must do to take in a sufficient amount to help us. We need to eat the right foods and eat foods that have not been altered by processing (thus potentially destroying the essential fatty acids).

The dosage

It is suggested that we need 300 and 400mg of both EPA and DHA a day to remain healthy, and higher levels during growth periods. So children, who are constantly growing, need a good supply. We also need more when things have gone wrong, as in the case of a child with developmental delay. The manufacturers of supplement capsules recommend, as do Tinsley House Clinic, a doubling of the normal dose for the first three months of supplementation. (See the individual manufacturers' recommended dosage on the packaging.)

DID YOU KNOW?

It is thought that 25 percent of the dry weight—with all the water taken out—of the brain is DHA (docosahexaenoic acid/omega-3). This is why it is so important to make sure we get enough of this essential omega-3.

WE ALL NEED GOOD FATS

A deficiency of fats will produce symptoms that may include:
- learning and behavioral difficulties
- poor short-term memory
- poor concentration
- clumsiness
- visual disturbances
- recurrent infections
- allergies
- constant thirst
- itchy dry eyes
- raised cholesterol
- raised blood pressure
- inflammatory diseases such as arthritis

The benefits of supplementing your diet include:
- increased concentration
- brain functioning at optimum
- better for your eyes, skin and joints
- mental alertness
- better ability to cope with emotional challenges
- better ability to do schoolwork

Fish and fish oils are a rich source of omega-3, notably the cold-water fish such as herring, mackerel, salmon and tuna. How often are these fish on your children's plate? These fish need to be on the menu, ideally, three times a week for your children to get the right amount through their diet. I'd say that very few of us manage to do this.

If your children can't eat fish the alternative is flaxseed oil, widely available in health-food shops, either as capsules or in liquid form that can be used in food preparation.

The omega-6 family is based on linoleic acid. It is converted during metabolic processes within the body to gamma-linolenic acid (GLA) and is found in its highest concentrations within the human body in the brain. Our brain needs this fat to function.

Omega-6 is found in sunflower oil, corn oil, sesame oil, hemp oil, pumpkin oil, soybean oil, walnut oil, wheatgerm oil and evening primrose oil. It is ultimately converted to prostaglandins—hormone-like molecules—that regulate such things as inflammation, blood pressure, and heart, gut and kidney functions. These come either in capsules, or liquid form to be used in cooking.

Omega-3 and omega-6 essential fatty acids are best consumed in a ratio of about three omega-6 for every one of omega-3. Both are available in capsule form from health-food shops. However, as omega-6 is found in so many foods, obtaining these levels should not be a problem providing you are having a reasonably well-balanced diet.

GLOSSARY OF TERMS

Essential fatty acids—Omega-3 and omega-6. They are critical for good health but cannot be made in the body. Therefore, it is essential that they are obtained from the food we eat. Omega-3 is commonly deficient in our diets.

Polyunsaturated fatty acids (PUFA)—Name of the group containing omega-3 and omega-6

Omega-3—There are three subtypes, explained below: EPA, DHA and ALA

EPA—Eicosapentaenoic acid. Source—oily fish and offal

DHA—Docosahexaenoic acid. Source—oily fish

> ALA—Alpha-linolenic acid. Source—dark-green leafy vegetables and flaxseed oil
>
> LA—Linoleic acid. Source—vegetables, fruit, nuts, grain and seeds

Benefits

Cell Membrane

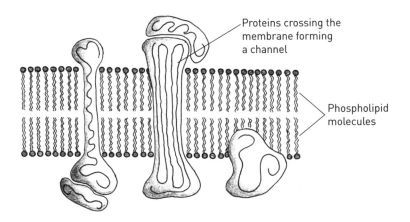

Phospholipids are needed by every cell in the body as it is a key building block of the cell membrane. The amount of phospholipids taken in through food is declining, as the foods rich in phospholipids are not eaten as often as they once were.

In the 1980s eggs had a really bad press in the UK, since which time many people have been reluctant to include them in their everyday diet. Egg yolks and such foods as liver, kidney, heart and brains are rich sources of phospholipids, but these old-fashioned recipes are no longer widely eaten.

Contrary to popular belief, eggs do not raise blood-cholesterol levels or predispose you to heart disease. In fact, properly fed free-range chickens provide eggs that in terms of phospholipids are super-foods.

Lecithin, a phosphoglyceride, is an alternative source of

phospholipids. It is produced by the liver if the diet is good, and is composed mostly of B-vitamins, phosphoric acid, choline, linoleic acid and inositol. Strangely, although it is a fatty substance, it is also a fat emulsifier—it helps to breaks down fats—and is considered vital to the health of the circulatory system.

LECITHIN

- Lecithin is a fat made of choline and inositol.
- Good sources are soybean, egg yolks, grains, fish, beans and peanuts.
- It is a rich source of choline, needed by the body to produce acetylcholine, an important neurotransmitter.

Similarly, phosphatidyl serine is vital to both brain-cell structure and function. It plays an important role in our neurotransmitter systems, metabolism levels of the brain and maintaining nerve synapses (connections) in the brain.

Traditionally our greatest source of serine came from eating offal, but diets have changed and liver and kidneys might not go down too well with the children these days. This presents a particular problem as it would appear that phosphatidyl serine levels naturally decline with age—though unproven this has a possible implication for dementia (see Chapter 13)—and this may be advanced if dietary levels are reduced in the first place, that is, if we don't eat them when we are children.

Fats are essential for the brain's communication system

Before summing up what all this means in terms of the symptoms of developmental delay syndrome, we need to consider the brain's communication system in some detail.

A neuron can talk to other neurons either directly by electrical stimulation at what are called gap-junctions, or indirectly by the use of neurotransmitters that can cross the gap (synapse) between two neurones and pass a message on. The neuron needs to be in optimum condition to work effectively, and you can achieve this by following this dietary advice.

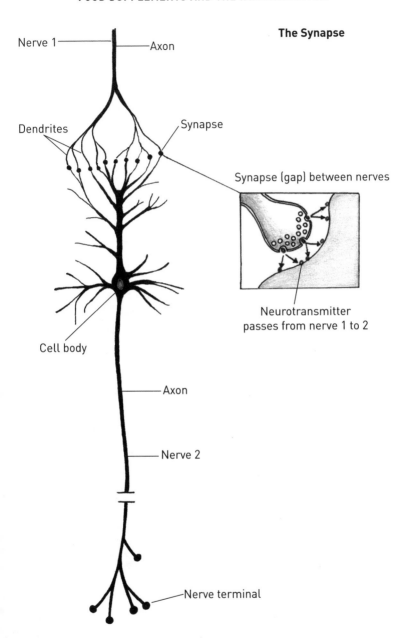

Zinc sulfate

For some time now we have all been made aware of the importance of essential fatty acids to the development of our children's nervous systems. Now new research has shown that adding zinc sulfate enhances the action of these essential fatty acids, both in the building of the cell wall and in the manufacture of certain neurotransmitters.

The authors of one study stated:

> Zinc supplements may exert their positive effects by helping to regulate the function of the neurotransmitter dopamine. Dopamine signaling, which has been implicated in causing symptoms of ADHD, is believed to play an important role in the feelings of pleasure and reward.

This "pleasure area" is thought to be the main reason why so many children with developmental delay syndromes crave junk food and establish a carbohydrate diet for themselves, thus fueling their addiction. This seeming addiction to sugars and the high intake of food additives complicates and perpetuates the underlying neurophysiological disorder.

SCIENTIFIC PROOF

Recent studies, notably in Teheran, have looked at the effects of providing 55mg of zinc sulfate a day to children with ADHD. The results indicate that zinc sulfate at this dosage level is as effective, if not more so, than prescribing Ritalin®.

Currently, based on research from different parts of the globe, it is suggested that adding zinc sulfate to the daily administration of omega-3 and omega-6 (essential fatty acids) enhances the action of Ritalin® or may be used in its place.

This is very exciting news as at present there is a great deal of concern about the use of Ritalin® and the long-term effects it may have. As zinc is a normal part of our diet in red meat, fish, poultry, oysters, mussels and some beans, and as far as we know has no side effects apart from a metallic taste in the mouth and/or nausea in some cases, this may prove to be a valuable aid in the treatment of conditions such as ADHD.

It is readily available: for instance, Nature's Way have their own brand of zinc capsule (30mg). All the research to date has used 55mg a day, so it is difficult to suggest a dosage. At present I am using common sense and suggesting a dosage related to body weight until such time as more research has been conducted and a formula for dosage established. I suggest that you seek advice from your pharmacist on what dosage your child should be taking if you are unsure.

BENEFITS FOR THE IMMUNE SYSTEM

Toward the end of the consultation and before the examination process I always question the parents concerning their child's medical history. For this I provide fixed prompts—illnesses, operations, broken bones, being knocked unconscious, any stitches, accidents, knocks, bangs, falls or crashes. Once these questions are answered, I then ask specifically about allergies and recurrent infections. Again I provide prompts—eczema, asthma or middle ear infections.

When I first started asking these questions I was fascinated by the number of times parents would say, "Oh yes, David had tubes." Now I suppose I've almost come to expect it, and I am amazed that no one else seems to have put two and two together and realized why this is. Put simply, the immune system—our built-in defense system against germs—has to have an executive in control and where do you think that is? You guessed it—in the brain. The two sides of the brain have slightly different functions in terms of that executive control, but both need to be working at near full capacity for the system to work.

We have already discussed the new wave of brain development that goes on four months after birth (see Chapter 4) and it would seem that when this development goes awry not only does the child run the risk of developmental delay, but also an immune system that either does not kick in as quickly as it should or else runs out of control.

Every child that visits Tinsley House Clinic is given a set of hearing tests and, if anything is wrong, the child's hearing is monitored at every visit until the results are normal. As the machines print out the results both in graph form and in figures, the parents can monitor the progress their child is making objectively in terms of their general health as well as the overall improvement in their developmental delay.

Also, using an otoscope (the device doctors use to probe your ear) with a built-in video camera means that the parents and the child get the opportunity—which many kids love—to look at and through the eardrum. As often as not, before the start of treatment you can see the telltale signs in the middle ear. For older children this, together with the other tests, shows the scars left by a history of repeated infections.

What I often see after only the first two or three treatments, and with the child on the Eating Plan, is that parents remark on the fact that their child no longer has a constantly runny nose or that they haven't gone down with the chest infection that they always get at this time of year. Parents see a rapid improvement in their child's skin or comment on a reduced use of the inhaler and their child's ability to run about without getting out of breath. In fact, if you simply measure the child's chest expansion with a tape before treatment and afterwards, there is generally a significant improvement in expansion and therefore the ability to breathe correctly.

It is essential to realize that not only will dyslexia, dyspraxia, ADD, etc., go hand in hand, never appearing in isolation, but that many childhood afflictions can accompany them. The child's brain is struggling and as a result the body is struggling too.

11

THE TINSLEY HOUSE CLINIC
14-DAY EATING PLAN

In previous chapters I've explained that there are very good reasons for making sure that your child eats the best possible diet that you can provide for them.

There is a lot of everyday evidence—that is, how parents see their child's behavior change after eating certain foods—as well as research revealing the negative effects of sugary, additive-loaded food. With all that we now know, surely we cannot carry on feeding these foods to our children.

As well as the learning and behavioral problems we've discussed in this book, there are other reasons to reconsider your child's diet. There is a huge increase in obesity in children, particularly in Western countries. This can lead to all sorts of health problems for a child as well as more serious health problems in later life.

Many food manufacturers and fast-food outlets have realized that parents are becoming more aware and concerned about their children's diets and they like to be seen to be responding to this problem. As their commercial interests are paramount, it is best not to rely on them to do the right thing but to take action for your child yourself. Make their diet as healthy as possible, read food labels to insure you're not buying food laden with additives, sugar and salt, and you will reap the benefits, with a healthier, happier child.

Let's go through the three main meals of the day and how they may affect your child's behavior and their ability to concentrate.

Then we'll introduce the 14-day Eating Plan for a healthy new start for your child.

BREAKFAST

It is vitally important to get breakfast right. The quality of your child's breakfast will help or hinder them at kindergarten and in grade school. A healthy breakfast will help your child to concentrate and avoid the behavioral problems associated with sugar highs and lows. A bad breakfast will produce a child who cannot concentrate or behave appropriately in class, as well as bringing on additive-induced mood swings.

LUNCH

If your child is at home with you, or has packed lunches, it is all under your control. You can make sure that they get the right sort of good food that they need.

What you need to do is to insure that your child gets protein and vegetables at lunchtime, followed by some fruit.

If you make packed lunches for your child and you're worried about having the time to start the 14-day plan (which may involve more cooking and/or a different routine from what you're used to) perhaps it might be worth looking at your child's school dinners. If they do offer healthy school dinners then give yourself a break and put your child on them. At least then you won't have to think about lunch and, instead, you can focus your energy on preparing healthy and interesting breakfasts and dinners.

If your child has kindergarten or school dinners it will be more difficult to control their diet but certainly not impossible. You may need to enlist the assistance of the school nurse or nutritionist if there is one on staff to make sure your child makes the right choices. Give them a list of things that your child can and can't eat. If you explain why you are so concerned about their diet I'm sure you'll be able to get their help.

KEEP TRACK OF WHAT THEY EAT WHEN THEY'RE NOT WITH YOU:

- Ask your day-care provider or babysitter to tell you what your child has eaten each day.

DINNER

This can often be the most difficult meal of all as it is the time of day when the child is most likely to be overexcited or tired (often they're overexcited *because* they're tired) and so less inclined to eat.

If you get breakfast and lunch right there will be less pressure on at dinner time to get your child to eat a full dinner. The meals suggested here are things that your child should like: often they're comforting, always they're tasty. If they are often tired after kindergarten or school, then they'll love the comfort food such as chicken pot pie, firm favorites like mini-burgers, spaghetti and meatballs, or even soup (which doesn't even have to be chewed).

Make it easy for them by offering sliced apple or sliced banana for dessert and a small fork. Use any techniques like this that you can think of to lessen the likelihood of them refusing to eat because they are tired or can't be bothered.

MEETING RESISTANCE

If your child won't eat the healthy food, persist in offering it to them without pressure.

For instance if they hate peas, don't give up, offer them again and cooked in a different way. They may hate plain boiled peas but perhaps they'll eat peas in chicken pot pie or with pasta and ham (see the recipes at the back of the book) or slightly disguised and flavored, say with grated Parmesan cheese on top.

Do offer treats for eating the new healthier diet but make the treats non-food items (see page 143 for some ideas).

Even the most hardened junk addicts can be won over with persistence and clever presentation of food.

ORGANIC IS BEST

Wherever you can afford to, buy free-range or organic foods. Even though these will almost certainly be more expensive than conventionally farmed foods they may not cost too much more than pre-prepared and packaged versions.

The most important place to spend your money if you can only afford a few organic items is to prioritize in this order: meat and chicken, then eggs, and last of all vegetables.

With non-organic fruit and vegetables, wash them thoroughly before you use them.

Typical examples of a child's daily diet showing the good and the bad

Breakfast
    Good—Eggs and bacon
    Bad—Cereals with high sugar content and added sugar, and white toast

Mid-morning
    Good—an apple
    Bad—potato chips with food additives, cookies and/or chocolate

Lunch
    Good—a properly cooked school lunch or sandwiches
    Bad—burger and fries, candy

Mid-afternoon
    Good—fruit or raw vegetables
    Bad—cookies, cake, potato chips, candy

Evening meal
    Good—home-cooked meat/fish and vegetables
    Bad—pizza, pasta, desserts

Drinks
　　Good—water, some fruit juices, some cordials
　　Bad—sodas, drinks with high sugar content/aspartame/
　　stimulants

BENEFITS OF FOLLOWING THE 14-DAY EATING PLAN

This 14-day plan will give you lots of ideas of how to feed your child with the food that will help to improve or even treat their condition. It will take some adjustment to change your child's diet but it is worth it. For some of the food included in the eating plan you'll need a recipe, and recipes are included at the back of the book. They're quite straightforward and easy to make but if you have any problems send your query via the Tinsley House Clinic website (www.tinsleyhouseclinic.com).

You will see results in your child's behavior each day, and more significant results as soon as two weeks.

You will probably have some sort of revolt on your hands. Food is important to us all, but to a child who is "addicted" to sugars and carbohydrates, it is especially important. If you expect a reaction and prepare yourself for it, you'll get through it. Wherever possible in this chapter I will give tricks, hints and bribes to help you along the way.

Using rewards

Try being creative in the way you reward good eating. If, for instance, your children are into music, you can let them play a song very loudly, or maybe spend longer on a computer game, rather than giving them a sweet treat such as chocolate or fries. If you think about it, it is madness to reward good behavior with treats that contain sugar or additives: your child eats well, then you reward that good behavior with food that gives them a sugar or additive rush, which encourages hyper behavior, which may lead to them doing something naughty ... It doesn't make sense, does it? Nor is it fair on the child.

Make a star chart and use it for every meal—if they get enough stars for eating well by the end of the week, they will have earned the right to go out and choose a treat, such as a comic book or some stickers.

14-DAY FOOD PLAN SHOPPING LIST

You will need the following foodstuffs to follow the 14-day plan as laid out later.

Fruit and veg
Baby corn, broccoli, carrots, cucumber, bananas, apples, new potatoes, mushrooms, tangerines, yellow peppers, sweet potatoes, lettuce, garlic, onion, avocado, lemon, celery, melon, tomatoes
Whole nuts for snacks

Meat and fish
The best ground lamb or beef you can afford (organic or free range if possible)
Salmon, swordfish or other meaty fish
Good quality sausages
Bacon (organic if possible)
Lamb chops
Family pack of free-range or organic chicken pieces
Smoked mackerel—in the refrigerated section of your supermarket
Cod, salmon and shrimp for fish pie
Chicken livers if making paté (if not buy ready-made from supermarket)
Roasting meat of choice for Day 14 roast dinner

Fridge
Houmous
Yogurt
Parmesan cheese
Mozzarella cheese

Freezer
Frozen peas and corn for when in a hurry

Dry food
Oatmeal
Shredded Wheat
Eggs (one dozen, free range if possible)
Rice crackers
Sultanas
Dried fruit: apricots, apples, papaya or bananas (organic
    if possible)—experiment and find their
    favorites
Honey
Wholemeal spaghetti—fusilli (spirals)
Brown rice
Popcorn—unpopped
Tacos
Olive oil (best oil to use)
Can of black olives
Can of tomatoes
Can of borlotti or kidney beans
Can of tuna

Bakery
Good brown or seeded bread such as Orowheat or Roman Meal
    (it is expensive but kids will have less of it), kept in the
    fridge to keep it fresher
Wholemeal pitta bread—can be stored in freezer and taken out
    as needed

Drinks
These should be good quality only, without sugar or other
    additives, e.g. smoothies (check for sugar/aspartame
    content). Or make them at home
Pure fruit juices—all supermarkets now have small cartons of
    organic orange and apple juice, which comes without
    added sugar, so use these for school

At home give water as often as possible or add water to the larger cartons for a diluted juice drink

Snacks
Rice crackers
Dried apricots, apples, bananas, papaya or sultanas
Walnuts or almonds, in the shell (kids have fun cracking them)

HELP, MY KIDS LOVE WHITE BREAD? I CAN'T STOP THEM FROM HAVING IT . . .

It is vitally important to find a bread your children like that is also healthy (one that is not white, spongy and lethal in terms of raising their blood-sugar levels). A company called Orowheat make fantastic bread, full of seeds and grains, which won't give them a sugar high and will help them go to the bathroom regularly.

They will get used to the change. If they really resist, continue to give them their usual spreads (however sugary they are) so that the change is not too drastic for them (changing or avoiding sugary jams and other sweet spreads can be tackled later).

Another trick is to cut the bread into interesting shapes to distract them from the change.

THE 14-DAY EATING PLAN

Day One—Monday

Breakfast: Scrambled egg with wholegrain toast

Snack: Rice cracker
         Banana

Lunch: A picking lunch gives your child a sense of choice, and could consist of: pieces of good-quality ham, carrot sticks, chunks of cucumber, olives, baby tomatoes and an apple—anything that is healthy in fact.

Dinner: Salmon or cod with boiled new potatoes and peas or corn

Day Two—Tuesday

Breakfast:	Sausages and mushrooms
Snack:	Home-popped popcorn
	Tangerine
Lunch:	Boiled egg with funny face drawn on with felt tip
	Houmous in wholemeal pitta bread cut into strips
	Strips of crunchy orange pepper
	An apple or other fruit
Dinner:	Lamb chops—meat on a stick like the cavemen ate
	Peas, carrots and mashed potato

Day Three—Wednesday

Breakfast:	Oatmeal sweetened with honey and topped with grated apple (grated apple easily stirs in if you need to hide it)
Snack:	Melon smiles (see recipes) or rice crackers
Lunch:	Beans (borlotti or red kidney in the can) with tuna (if there's any left over save the tuna for pizza on Day Five), finely chopped onion, a squeeze of lemon juice and a dash of olive oil
Dinner:	Spiral (fusilli) pasta with tomato sauce
	Hidden vegetable pasta sauce containing carrots, celery, onions, garlic, tomatoes and topped with freshly grated Parmesan cheese

(Tip: make a huge batch of sauce and freeze in ice-cube trays, three cubes per child—this saves you time too)

Day Four—Thursday

Breakfast:	Boiled egg and bread strips
Snack:	Small box of sultanas
Lunch:	Houmous wraps
	Baby corn, baby carrots
	Melon smiles
Dinner:	Home-made mini-burgers with ground organic beef, grated apple, sweet potato and finely chopped onion all concealed in the burger
	Serve with brown rice (not a bun) and a little tomato ketchup

Day Five—Friday

Breakfast: Shredded Wheat topped with sliced bananas

Snack: Raisins

Lunch: Leftover mini-burgers, mini-corns, mini-carrots, apple, olives

Dinner (Friday night treat): Healthy pizza, wholegrain pitta bread with tomato sauce, mozzarella cheese, and tuna and olives on top

Tailor the toppings to suit your child's taste—let them put their own toppings on to include them in cooking, get them interested in food in general and, more importantly, what they are eating

Day Six—Saturday

Breakfast: Bacon and tomato sandwiches

Snack: Dried apricots, dried apples or bananas

Try your child on all of them to find their favorite

Lunch: Brown rice salad with chopped tomato, cucumber, pieces of chopped bacon left over from breakfast

Favorite cheese grated on top

Try giving each ingredient separately rather than mixing in together (as you would do for an adult salad) so that they can see what is in their food and don't get any surprises

Dinner: Free-range or organic oven-roasted chicken drumsticks with broccoli and home-made fries (see recipe)

Day Seven—Sunday

Breakfast: Baked beans with wholegrain toast triangle scoops

Snack: Small pot of sultanas

Lunch: Leftover chicken drumsticks and cucumber and carrot sticks, baby tomatoes

Chunk of their favorite cheese—Cheddar or Parmesan

Tangerine

Dinner: Spaghetti and meatballs (wholemeal pasta)

Make enough meatballs to have leftovers for lunch tomorrow

GOOD SNACKS:

- Any fruit your child wants—lots of fruit is sweet enough to keep kids happy, especially grapes and melon, nectarines and strawberries
- Rice cakes, oatcakes (plain or with avocado or banana "smashed" onto them with a drizzle of honey to sweeten)
- Dried fruit (try in small quantities until they are used to it)
- Home-popped popcorn

Day Eight—Monday in a rush

Breakfast: Shredded Wheat in winter

Fruit salad in summer—experiment with toppings: crunchy nuts, dried fruit and yogurt

Toasted almond flakes (toppings can be kept in small Tupperware pots and children can sprinkle their own on)

Snack: Fruit of their choice

Lunch: Mini-meatballs (left over from yesterday's dinner)

Cherry tomatoes

Baby corn

Olives

Apple

Dinner: Tacos with shredded chicken and salad including lettuce, tomatoes, grated Cheddar cheese and sliced avocado

Day Nine—Tuesday

Breakfast: Scrambled eggs and beans

Snack: Fruit, dried fruit or a rice cracker

Lunch: Home-made chicken-liver paté sandwiches (or a good-quality shop-bought paté)

Baby corn, carrot sticks, olives

Tangerine

Dinner: Swordfish/cod/haddock (a steak of fish) with home-made fries and peas or broccoli

> ## YOU GET WHAT YOU PAY FOR
>
> Cheaper baked beans usually contain more sugar to give them more flavor.

Day Ten—Wednesday

Breakfast: Homemade paté on toast (left over from yesterday) OR
Shredded Wheat with sliced banana on top
Snack: Any fruit
Lunch: Boiled egg with silly message on it in felt tip (or a face if the child can't read)
Small pot of houmous with dipping veg, carrot sticks, peppers, cucumbers and mushrooms
Dinner: Spaghetti Bolognese (with loads of veg)
Wholemeal pasta

Day Eleven—Thursday

Breakfast: Sausages and eggs (however you want them)
Cook the whole pack of sausages for leftovers for lunch tomorrow
Snack: Banana
Lunch: Good-quality bread sandwich with filling of the child's choice
Selection of favorite veg sticks
Piece of cheese
Apple
Dinner: Fisher-girl/boy's pie
Cod, haddock, or salmon in a cheesy sauce topped with mashed potato

Day Twelve—Friday

Breakfast: Boiled egg and bread strips
Snack: Banana, popcorn
Lunch: Sausages (from Day Eleven breakfast) with the child's favorite veg sticks and seasonal fruit of their choice
Dinner: Chilli con carne and rice, grated cheese to go on top

Day Thirteen—Saturday

Breakfast: Scrambled eggs and smoked mackerel (flake the fish with a fork to break it up)

Snack: Apple, tangerine, rice crackers

Lunch: Chilli con carne in pitta pocket (left over from last night's dinner)

Dinner: Fishcakes
Vegetables—corn or salad

Day Fourteen—Sunday

Breakfast: A treat for making it through: pancakes with banana and honey filling

Snack: Apple, tangerine or dried fruit

Lunch: Good-quality fresh soup (found in the refrigerator section at the supermarket) or, if you can, home-made

Dinner: Roast dinner: lamb or chicken with roast potatoes, carrots, peas, broccoli

---

YOU GET WHAT YOU PAY FOR

- It is worth having a close look at jam labels to check their contents. Some jams contain more sugar to make up for a lack of fruit.

- Look for reasonably cheap, large family packs of free-range chicken. It really is worth paying for this, as the taste is far better and it isn't mass-produced, battery chicken which sits squashed up all day long.

  If you can afford organic, even better—the meat should be free of antibiotics especially if you buy it from a reliable butcher rather than a supermarket.

Rocket fuel—Christopher, aged seven

*Christopher flew down from Scotland with his mother to see me. It was not a happy meeting as Christopher was **hyperactive** with a capital H, literally bouncing off the walls. During the consultation* *process the roots of his problems became evident, but when we finally discussed Christopher's diet it became all too clear that he was addicted to sugar and took enough fuel on board each day to put a rocket into orbit. His poor diet in combination with liberal helpings of assorted bad food additives and aspartame meant his developing brain was struggling to function, let alone mature.*

Following a harrowing examination (for me) Christopher was sent on his way with a set of simple exercises to carry out each day and a detailed healthy diet plan to follow, which included a daily double dose of omega-3 and omega-6. One week later his mother called to ask if the treatment should be working yet. Before I could answer she informed me that it was and that Christopher was a different boy: calm, settled, quieter and a joy to be with.

ADHD—Jimmy, aged nine

Jimmy's mother brought him to see me having reached the end of her rope. The final straw came when Jimmy was excluded from school, at just nine years old.

*Both in the classroom and at home Jimmy was out of control, being **unable to keep still**, having **violent outbursts** and periods of **destructive behavior**. On further questioning it became clear that, apart from the **hyperactivity**, Jimmy had aspects of Tourette's syndrome. So far this had been missed and the impression given by his mother was that Jimmy was considered to be a bad boy from the wrong part of town.*

*Jimmy had attained all the developmental milestones on time apart from **bladder control** at night, which was only attained at seven years of age. There was, however, a family history of what Jimmy's mother called **behavioral problems** on the father's side of the family.*

*At about seven years of age Jimmy had suddenly become disobedient and over the period of the next six months had become **disruptive** at school, **violent** and wantonly **destructive** at home. He was slow getting dressed, had difficulty with **fine motor skills** and had an appalling **short-term memory**.*

*Watching Jimmy was all that was necessary to see the extent of his problems. He had a left-sided **facial tic**, **involuntary movements** of his neck and the habit of letting the odd mild expletive out when he could no longer keep his head and neck still. Jimmy had aspects of ADHD, dyspraxia, dyslexia, OCD and Tourette's syndrome, and* *was clearly struggling to maintain control, which accounted for his extremely low level of self-esteem. During conversations we had later on following treatment, Jimmy didn't mention the words depression or suicide, but it was evident from what he did say that his life had been a living hell.*

A very strict diet was started straight away, which as expected exacerbated his behavior for a few days before he started to settle. However, it soon became clear that Jimmy was addicted to sugars and it took a great deal of cooperation, not to mention bribery, between his mother and the school to stop him selling his healthy packed lunch so that he could buy candy.

Once Jimmy decided to stick to the diet, and his mother became an additive expert, his behavior changed dramatically and the violent outbursts came to an end. He responded very well to treatment and on his fourth visit to the clinic there were no signs of involuntary movements and his mother stated that they now had a totally different boy. This latter aspect was reflected in his school reports, with comments concerning not only his improved behavior but also his academic achievements.

Dyspraxia—Tania, aged nine

Tania's passage into the world was not an easy one. The plan was, due to anticipated birthing problems, that a trial labor would be started with the option of a caesarean section should it prove necessary. In the end, Tania was delivered by an assisted birth during which her skull was fractured.

*She was described by her mother as having been a "floppy baby" and as a result of this spent the first two weeks of her life in the Special Care Unit. Tania was a quiet baby. She **did not sit unassisted** until nine months, **did not crawl** and **did not walk** until twenty-two months. Her **first words** did not appear until fourteen months and she **could not string two words** together until nearly three years of age, preferring **pre-declarative signing** (pointing to an object when you don't have the name for it).*

*Tania was a **slow learner**, had problems with both gross and fine **motor skills**, took everything said to her **literally** and could never understand a joke. **Hyperactivity** both at home and at school had become a serious concern as her behavior disrupted the class and prevented learning.*

On examination she maintained a head tilt to the left, swayed dramatically once her eyes were closed during the Rhomberg's test and consistently undershot on the left when attempting the Finger to Nose test. On muscle testing, weakness was present on the right side of her body, most noticeably in the small muscles of the hands and feet. She was grossly dyspraxic and demonstrated textbook dysdiadochokinesia. The cranial nerve testing showed up problems with both her right and left eyes, beyond what would be picked up by an optician. She also had problems with her blood pressure and her hearing.

Following her first treatment at the clinic, a problem with her right eye responded immediately. Tania was put on a strict diet for two weeks that included reduced carbohydrates, no food additives and no artificial sweeteners. For the first three days of the diet Tania's behavior worsened, with aggressive outbursts and tantrums every five minutes. As if by magic, from day four onwards, her level of activity reduced along with the aggression and tantrums. At the end of the two-week trial period Tania's parents were convinced of the need to stick with the diet.

Following an eye test at the opticians, Tania was prescribed glasses and with her new 20/20 vision was able to start a computer-generated program designed to improve her right eye.

After six months of treatment (which only involved five actual treatments) Tania was talking normally, behaving normally and was rapidly catching up with her schoolwork. Her diet is still monitored closely and she takes omega-3 and omega-6 daily together with zinc sulfate. Obviously, it will take some time for Tania to catch up on all the schooling she has missed, but with a little extra help both at home and at school, this should not pose a problem.

When last seen at the clinic it was difficult to imagine that this was the same girl, particularly when she caught me with a joke that I really should have seen coming.

ADHD—Samantha, aged six

Samantha, aged six years, was brought to see me by her parents, who were reaching their breaking point. They described her as a total nightmare.

As a baby she had **not fed well** and was late attaining the developmental milestones for **sitting, walking** and **talking**. She **did not crawl** and was described as a **bottom-shuffler**.

From about twenty-one months she had become **hyperactive** both *in the home and at daycare. She was constantly noisy, **easily distracted**, had a poor **short-term memory**, was a **messy eater** and had a tendency to be **destructive** for no apparent reason.*

*Her early years were peppered with **constant ear infections**, outbreaks of **eczema** and **asthma attacks**. She'd had **numerous accidents**, which her parents attributed to the fact that she always seemed to **move too quickly** and as a result was very **clumsy**.*

*On questioning the mother concerning diet a very familiar picture appeared. Because the child was a **fussy eater** the mother in despair had given her whatever she would eat on the basis that anything is better than nothing. Unfortunately, in this situation the child insidiously dictates the menu and the parent obliges, often by providing endless carbohydrate-based meals, snack foods and sodas.*

Samantha was no exception and when her mother provided me with a list of all food and drink consumed over a two-week period, over 80 percent of the items on the list had to be eliminated and replaced with food and drinks free of additives and low in sugars.

For the next three days Samantha's behavior deteriorated and her parents despaired. Then remarkably, on the morning of the fourth day, the parents were blessed with a totally different child. Samantha had slowed down, ate her meal calmly without making a mess and was a joy to be with. Following five treatments her parents reported that she continued to eat without making a mess, was concentrating better at school, was well behaved, was speaking more slowly and making perfect sense.

When re-tested all her neurological findings showed a marked improvement including the hearing test—tympanometry—which showed a clear change.

Falling behind at school—Lauren, aged eight

Eight-year-old Lauren was brought to see me by her parents as over the past four school terms her school reports showed that she was struggling to keep up—the final blow came when they had been informed at a recent parents' evening that she would be held back a grade if the decline continued.

Lauren was a very pleasant, polite, calm young lady who remained seated throughout the consultation process and answered all the questions put to her by me and responded with good humor all the while I teased her.

There was no family history of learning or behavioral problems, the pregnancy and delivery were all a mother could ask for, and she was only slightly delayed in sitting, walking and talking. There were no major signs of developmental delay other than a hint of **dyspraxia**. *On examination there were further signs of dyspraxia and several clues that the right prefrontal cortex was struggling.*

During the consultation I had asked specifically about the family diet and it was abundantly clear that, due to family pressures borne of a hectic adult work schedule, the bulk of the food consumed was processed, pre-prepared, convenience meals. The children drank sugar-loaded drinks ad infinitum together with the inevitable aspartame that sodas contain.

The treatment plan was as follows:

- *no junk food*
- *no bad food additives*
- *no artificial sweeteners*
- *reduce bad fats, carbohydrates and sugars*
- *monitor salt content*
- *add omega-3 and omega-6 (double dose for three months, then a maintenance dose)*
- *parental education—healthy eating*
- *establish a daily routine for homework and sleeping*
- *simple daily exercises designed to stimulate the cerebellum*

Within two weeks Lauren's energy levels soared and so did her schoolwork. She was able to concentrate, to stay focused and to last the day out without flagging. At bedtime she was healthily tired and in the mornings refreshed and alert. When reassessed after two months she was discharged from treatment, while her parents were charged with supplying me with her school reports.

This was a case of a very minor form of developmental delay where the struggling brain was hampered by a combination of poor diet and increasing workload. Once the balance was adjusted Lauren never looked back.

Food for thought—Bridget, aged eight

Bridget flew in with her mother from the south of France to my clinic in the south of England. As a general rule I prefer to treat children *that are a little closer to hand, but in this case I need not have worried. At consultation a very typical story began to unfold. There was a family history of **learning problems** on both sides of the family, Bridget had had a **slightly difficult birth**, her milestones were a little delayed, she had had endless **middle-ear problems**, **eczema** and had been mildly **asthmatic**. Since starting school she had not coped too well and now was falling behind, becoming anxious, had frequent stomachaches in the morning which always settled quickly if kept off school, and was having accidents at night.*

*During the consultation process it became clear that Bridget was suffering from aspects of **dyslexia**, **dyspraxia**, **attention deficit**, some **hyperactivity**, some minor **obsessive behavior** and had a minor **facial tic**. She also had a poor **short-term memory**, a low level of self-esteem and hated herself when she wet the bed.*

*On examination she had minor **hearing problems**, could not bring her **eyes in toward her nose**, could not produce **coordinated movements** and had retained **primitive reflexes**.*

*When we discussed Bridget's diet it became very clear that big changes had to take place. She had always been a **fussy eater** but now survived almost entirely on cereals, junk food and sodas. Fortunately, Bridget was a very bright girl so I decided that my best chance of success was to get her to dictate the diet rather than having it imposed upon her by her parents. I tried to get across to her why it was important to eat a variety of different foods and that food additives upset a lot of children badly, slowing down the development of their brains.*

I sent Bridget and her mother back off to France with some strict dietary advice, some daily exercises to do and a computer-generated program to correct the minor visual problem. Two weeks later I received an e-mail from Bridget's mother saying that they had been unable to do the exercises or start the computer program as they had been away, but Bridget had adopted the dietary changes with a passion. Already a remarkable change had come over Bridget and she was exuding confidence, was bright, chatty and for the first time in ages had that joyous laughter every child should possess.

Bridget started her exercises, buckled down to the computer program and when seen by a colleague, who fortunately lived forty kilometers down the road, was making remarkable progress. The last time I spoke to my colleague Bridget was discharged from treatment and doing exceptionally well at school.

This eating plan has produced amazing results for Tinsley House Clinic patients. It can produce amazing results for your child too. Following this eating plan can heal any present difficulties and prevent future health problems for your child.

It may not be easy to get your child to stick to this plan, but neither is life easy now, for you or for your child who has a learning or behavioral difficulty. Set yourself the challenge of trying this eating plan for your child and you *will* see results. Check the Tinsley House Clinic website (www.tinsleyhouseclinic.com) if you have any problems with the plan and for further hints and tips on how to get your child eating healthily.

12

PARENTS

The Learning Disability Myth is a book aimed at parents who want to help their child, but this chapter is both *for* and *about* the parents of children who have developmental delay syndrome.

It is not just the children who suffer if they have DDS—the parents of those children suffer too. You won't need me to tell you this if you have a DDS child. Perhaps you've looked for help and support and found there is little to be had, or maybe you haven't really thought about how much it affects you and your family and you've just tried to get on with it.

At Tinsley House Clinic we know that parents need help, support and encouragement in order to help their child through treatment that will ultimately change their lives, and the lives of their families.

Often we tend to think of the immediate problem, the everyday effects, without considering the long-term effects for the child, or the difficulties that the child's behavior, or the extra attention they need, may have on family and classmates. In this chapter I will go into some detail about what the issues are for parents and provide some practical help with strategies to make changes. You'll also find in this chapter some case studies to illustrate how children, their parents and their families are affected.

Let's first look at parental stress. A side effect of DDS is that parents are under enormous stress and this can take many forms. One area that can cause serious stress is lack of sleep. Every parent has some sleepless nights after having children, but if disturbed nights are ongoing, continuing once the child is more than a year old, then the health and sanity of the parents can really begin to suffer. Sleep problems in a child can be a symptom of DDS and can be addressed with the same techniques I use to work on the brain. (See Chapter 6.)

The little boy who did not sleep—John, aged 21 months

John was seen at the clinic after a plea for help from his distressed, exhausted parents. At the consultation the need for help was patently obvious as his mother was about to have her second child in the next few weeks.

*John had been born at full-term but had suffered **fetal distress** due to possible ingestion/inhalation of meconium and had the umbilical cord around his neck. He was taken away immediately for suctioning, following which he appeared to be fine. Fine, that is, apart from being a very poor sleeper.*

*Over the months this situation had worsened so that he would not sleep during the day and at bedtime, even though appearing exhausted, would refuse to settle no matter what his parents did. If left alone he would start to scream hysterically and continue to the point that he would start vomiting. This naturally so distressed his parents that they were frightened to leave him. Even when he did eventually drop off to sleep he would awaken several times in the night with **night terrors**.*

*John had been **late attaining his developmental milestones** by a couple of months across the board, and yet while chatting to him and his parents I quickly came to realize that when he did attain these targets he was one of the most advanced children I had ever met. At 21 months he could put simple sentences together and had a vocabulary that would put much older children to shame. He was also very clearly a genius at getting his own way. As I talked to his parents, who were naturally concerned about getting him to sleep through the night, it rapidly became clear that this very smart young man was perfectly behaved by day providing he was getting exactly what he wanted. Now we had a completely different ball game.*

Having examined John as far as possible considering his age, I explained to the parents just what it was that I thought was happening. John was probably suffering a minor form of developmental delay, perhaps due to the fetal distress he had suffered. This, in a boy in particular, would tend to cause the right side of the brain to over-react to the normal events of the day and certainly of the night. The right side of the brain is the more primitive side and tends to deal with approach/withdrawal situations, that is, anything that is a potential danger to us. By day John made sure he had a parent at his side at all times and at night, when it is dark and the house makes its own sounds, he could not bear to be alone. It would only take an owl to hoot or the wind to howl and, even though exhausted, he would awaken in need of instant reassurance.

The treatment plan was twofold. One, start a simple exercise regime to stimulate the cerebellum and thereby the brain, and two, adopt simple old-fashioned toddler-training methods. By day tantrums would not be tolerated. If John behaved badly he would be told why he must behave, with the parent going down to floor level to do this. If this did not work he would be placed on a chair or a step where he must stay until he had settled down. The parents also had to learn that once they had said something it had to be carried out. Children need consistency, routine and most importantly to know in advance what is coming next.

His not being able to drop off to sleep was due to two simple things. Firstly, because the right side of the brain—which checks for danger—was not functioning normally John was frightened of everything, and secondly, because of this an area of his brain stem was overactive, keeping the brain awake. An undeveloped right brain needs routine, likes to know what is going to happen next and hates changes or surprises.

So while it was my job to deal with the underlying cause, the parents had to develop a regime to settle John well in advance of bedtime. Therefore, while he was finishing his evening meal he should be told he would soon be having his bath. While in the bath he should be told he would soon have to get out and be dried. While being dried he should be told he must then put on his pajamas and while doing this be told he must then get into bed ready for his bedtime story. Toward the end of his story he should be given his bottle and told that when the story is finished he will go to sleep until the morning. Once kissed goodnight he should be left to drift off.

John's treatment is still ongoing, but already he no longer has tantrums, sleeps through most nights and fortunately still has the most infectious giggle on the planet.

Another issue causing parental stress is discipline. Or lack of it, to be more precise. Parents can feel enormously guilty about their child's problems, and this seems to apply particularly to mothers, who wonder if they may have done something wrong in pregnancy or in raising their child. This guilt can have a bearing on how they treat the child.

Feeling guilty and overcompensating as a consequence can often leave siblings in the shade. How often have you said, "Sorry, I can't do that right now, I've got to see to your brother ..."

Discipline can break down. What I often see is that, because there is a problem with the child, parents can get into the habit of indulging them just to get through the day, and the night. Hand in hand with the right diet and treatment, we discuss discipline at Tinsley House, as it may need some adjustment within the family.

Here are some basic survival skills in discipline to give just some ideas for how to tackle it.

TEN DAILY STRATEGIES FOR COPING

1. Have a routine and stick with it for bathtime, bedtime and meals.
2. Remember that you are the parent and in charge.
3. Thinking that you are being kind giving candy is not a good idea.
4. Stick or carrot? Choose the most appropriate discipline technique for your child—some kids will respond to incentives and rewards, others to punishments and loss of rewards.
5. Be consistent.
6. Say what you mean and mean what you say.
7. Be kind but firm when necessary.
8. Curb all bad behavior from the start—if you are losing your temper on a regular basis, seek help.
9. Have fun with your kids—find time for them.
10. Give hugs each and every day.

Often, as the treatment begins to work or once it is complete, parents suddenly realize that changes do need to be made with their child's behavior, and it is a matter of changing how the child is disciplined. Perhaps they have got away with too much for too long.

To help with tackling discipline, I provide all of my clients with some basic but effective advice on discipline. This Parental Survival Plan will help you to "survive" living with a DDS child. It will also make life easier for siblings who may feel that the DDS child gets away with murder.

PARENTAL SURVIVAL PLAN

Job description
You are the parent/adult—they are the child. Beware of role reversal.

Never shout, but have two voices
Voice one: Firm—for giving instructions
Voice two: Melodious—for giving praise

Have routines and stick to them
Children with developmental delay do not like change or surprises. Therefore, have the week/day/hour planned ahead and always tell the child in advance just what is going to happen next.

Say what you mean and mean what you say
Once you have spoken there can be no going back, such as, "If you don't do as you are told I am going to…" and then you don't. No mixed messages.

Talk to the child at their level
That is both mentally and, more importantly, physically. Establish eye contact and get down to their level to talk to them, not from on high.

Zero tolerance
Bad behavior is not acceptable and not tolerated.

The "naughty spot"
Unacceptable behavior is punished by the child being told to sit on a stool or step for a prescribed period of time or until the behavior

changes. Do not send them to their room as this is not a punishment and may generate still further bad behavior or damage.

And, remember, love conquers all.

You might think that it's all very well for me to sit in my clinic talking about discipline. However, not only am I a father of four but I have also seen this work with my patients. The children respond so well to being given firmer boundaries that you'll be glad you made changes. The most frequent comment I hear from parents is "I wish I'd tried this earlier."

You can judge for yourself how this plan works in practice when you read the following case studies.

A copycat ADHD case—Simon, aged five

I had previously treated Mark, an eight-year-old boy with supercharged ADHD, and had been asked by his mother if I would take a look at his younger brother Simon. She was concerned that with a family history of behavioral problems on the father's side Simon, who had always been active, was now going the way of his brother with full-blown ADHD. Obviously the family history was in place but there any similarities ceased. With Simon the pregnancy and delivery had been textbook, he had attained all his developmental milestones on time, and on examination I could find nothing wrong with him.

At this point an all-too-familiar pattern started to unfold. He had always been active, but not hyperactive until he reached an age where he could observe his older brother, noticed that he always got his own way, and obviously thought this was how to behave. When I chatted things over with the parents out of earshot of the boys I could see the realization flooding over them. Simon had done what we all do as we grow up and had mimicked the behavior of his big brother, obviously not realizing that this was not normal acceptable behavior.

The solution was simple, but to put it in place took a great deal of determination on the part of his parents and a not inconsiderable contribution from his now much calmer big brother. The parents were given a copy of my Parental Survival Plan, wished "Good luck" and told to ring me within two weeks. Following five days and nights of hell Simon had finally given in and, much to his surprise, found himself considerably happier and surrounded by a close and loving family.

Whatever your view on discipline, something that is clear is that it has to start at home. An ICM poll commissioned by digital channel Teachers' TV shows that teachers agree with this statement. This survey of teachers found that they believe that parents are the biggest contributing factor to disciplinary problems in classrooms. In fact:

- More than 80 percent of teachers said they thought lack of parental support or control was to blame for behavioral problems.
- More than 50 percent thought parents should be made to stay at home to look after suspended children.
- 19 percent of teachers said they spent 10 percent of their time in class dealing with disruptive children.
- 72 percent backed a zero-tolerance policy.

Treatment working but behavior not improving—Joe, aged six

Joe and his older sister Sophie were both adopted, fortunately by two of the most wonderful human beings on the planet, and yet while Sophie was any parent's dream come true, Joe was a serious challenge, to say the least. When Joe was six, they all arrived at the clinic, minus any family history of course, but with a tale of woe that had me deeply concerned within minutes.

Joe had apparently been late sitting unaided (around eight or nine months), had crawled but did not attempt to walk until he was seventeen months. He was fine up until that point but once able to walk, all hell broke loose, with him constantly on the move and always in trouble. Although he had started to speak in the first year his words were unclear and often incomprehensible. Unfortunately, he did not progress and ended up seeing a speech therapist, but to no great effect.

At six years of age he was still wet every night and, having been dry by day at three years, regressed and would wet himself three or four times a day. More worryingly from my point of view, there were aspects of soiling.

At school a whole set of new problems arose, with Joe hitting and biting other children, not interacting with the children or staff, wandering off, being extremely loud, interrupting other children's work and banging doors or furniture continuously.

It had been noted at one point that Joe could not read other people's facial expressions or body language. This is a very important aspect of communication and although babies respond well to exaggerated facial expressions, its progress relies upon the development of the prefrontal cortex, notably the right.

On examination the extent of Joe's neurological problems became evident. This was clearly going to be an uphill struggle for me to come up with a treatment regime he could follow and one that his long-suffering parents could achieve. But Joe surprised us all, and after an initial reluctance took to his computer-generated programs like the proverbial duck to water. Over a period of weeks he improved beyond belief, showing remarkable improvement both when retested subjectively and objectively. There was only one problem—his behavior was if anything worse than ever.

Over the years Joe had got away with bloody murder, as everything he did was put down to his condition, and now his patterns of behavior were well and truly established. Having attained a particular level of improvement the time had come to have a quiet chat with Mum. So while Joe and Sophie played outside under the ever-watchful eye of their father, I broached the subject of parental control. The message must have struck home because the next day I received an e-mail asking if I thought that they should go on a behavior-management course. My suggestion was to follow the Parental Survival Plan strictly for two weeks, and if that didn't work to think again. Joe is no fool and within five days he had decided which side his bread was buttered on and began to comply. It will take time to change all the habits of his albeit short lifetime, but he will change given that time, and he will improve.

It is essential to realize that developmental delay and intelligence are two totally separate things and that behind all Joe's problems is a highly intelligent young man with a severely dented self-esteem, a high level of frustration and yet the potential to overcome all of this and succeed in life.

PARENTS WHO HAVE DDS

Sometimes treating the child's problem can be more complicated as it becomes evident that the parent or parents have problems too. Often these parents need support as they may have DDS themselves, and they may be unaware of it. And sometimes—and this may be hard to hear—a parent's behavior may be part of the problem, as we'll see in this next case study.

Tug of love?—Mark, aged eight

Mark's mother made an appointment for me to see him and then promptly canceled it. Within a week she had rebooked and was on the verge of canceling again when she changed her mind once more and went ahead with it. I expect parents to be a little apprehensive and nervous initially, but this lady was a nervous breakdown on legs. Her words came out as though fired from a machine gun, a right-sided facial tic punctuating the stressful story she was relating, and her hands constantly performed the most elaborated ritual of wringing movements. Every time her ex-husband's name was mentioned her head would make a sudden turn to the side to accompany an exaggerated facial tic.

We had been talking—she had been talking—for nearly twenty minutes and as yet there had been no mention of Mark, his problems or her concerns for him. At this point I took control of the situation and gently but firmly directed the conversation, now at last a dialog, toward the purpose of the visit. In a nutshell, Mark was beginning to **struggle at school**, *had become* **very emotional** *and had started* **wetting the bed** *on a nightly basis.*

The family history was dominated by her ex-husband's obsessive behavior, not only as a child but within the confines of the marriage, which she felt had contributed greatly to the marital breakdown. Mark had been born at full-term by natural delivery and, apart from the fact that the cord was around his neck, the birth had gone like clockwork. He had attained all his developmental milestones pretty well on time apart from gaining **bladder control**. *He was over three before being more or less dry by day and over five before becoming dry at night.*

He had always been a **nervous child**, *needing constant reassurance, and would frequently wake at night having had a bad dream. Calling out for his mother, he would enter his parent's bedroom and attempt to get into bed with his mother. His boarding-school-educated father considered this to be totally unnecessary behavior and would shout at Mark, ordering him back to bed.*

Mark had coped at school, clearly trying to the best of his ability, until the separation and divorce of his parents. From then on the bed-wetting returned and his schoolwork suffered badly. Not surprisingly under the circumstances, his mother found it increasingly difficult to cope with Mark and the situation was compounded by his father's almost Victorian attitude to his son's problems. This very soon produced a situation where Mark refused to visit his father when it was his weekend to have him, thus fueling further acrimonious accusations from him against his ex-wife.

The first thing Mark needed was a friend, and a very powerful alpha male at that. Well, we didn't have one of those, so he would have to make do with me. We arranged that he would call me a couple of times a week, supposedly to discuss how the treatment was going. In fact, we talked about everything except his treatment, with me slipping "That's really cool" into the dialog as often as I could. The treatment itself involved strict dietary changes, including no bad food additives and artificial sweeteners, plus the addition of omega-3 and omega-6 and some physical and computer-generated programs.

At first all went well. Within ten days the bed-wetting had stopped and his mother confirmed, what I had gathered from our chats on the phone, that his level of confidence was growing on a daily basis. In fact things were going so well that when his father insisted on having Mark for the weekend, he had agreed and gone off quite happily.

When he returned on the Sunday evening he was quiet, on edge and went straight to his room. His mother could get nothing from him other than, "It's nothing, leave me alone." That next day his father was on the phone to inform her that he had flushed the omega-3 and omega-6 down the toilet, wanted to know why she was starving him and wanted my telephone number as somebody needed to stop this quack messing up young kids.

Apparently, apart from flushing the omega capsules down the toilet, he had insisted on Mark eating good old-fashioned junk food, washed down with a well-known brand of soda, had ridiculed the exercise program and had taken away Mark's laptop, thus preventing him from doing his eye exercises. Needless to say, I had a very distraught mother on the phone in floods of tears asking what she could do.

Fortunately, the problem was taken out of our hands when Mark decided that he would not visit his father again if he had to eat junk *food and could not do his exercises. Faced with this ultimatum, eventually his father conceded and over a period of time not only helped Mark to stick to his regime, but started taking omega capsules himself. I am still awaiting the phone call.*

Most of the parents I see will do whatever it takes to help their child. What can be extremely disheartening is to see cases where it is obvious that the problem will persist because the parent cannot, or will not, do what is needed.

As we've discussed earlier, sometimes this is because the parent themself has DDS, or it may be that they simply find it too hard—for whatever reason—to make adjustments to their lives.

Great expectations—Oliver, aged eight

*Eight-year-old Oliver was brought to see me by his father. He had been born at full-term by natural delivery, had not suffered any fetal distress and took to the breast in no time. He attained his milestones on time until it came to **walking, which was late**—sixteen months—and **bladder control**, which was, to say the least, erratic both by day and night.*

*However, his father's concerns were with his education—he had already been dragged off for two separate assessments by educational psychologists and the father had made numerous visits to the school. Oliver was reluctant to read, was falling behind at school, did not do enough homework and clearly was a failure in his father's eyes. It was also very obvious that Oliver was a **nervous wreck**. If I turned in my chair he jumped out of his skin and before I could do the most basic of tests I had to explain exactly what it involved and reassure him that it would not hurt.*

I had questioned his father at length concerning any family history of learning or behavioral problems, but this was emphatically denied. However, I noticed at the time that there was not a hair out of place on this man and his clothing could have been brand new. Calling him immaculate would not have done him justice.

I was to learn over a relatively short period of time that this tidiness and order extended throughout his life and was being imposed upon his family. If there was a chance he might be late for an appointment he would call with a report on his location and the state of the traffic, and there would be numerous phone calls to confirm what Oliver should be doing treatment-wise or to ask if I thought he was on target and making satisfactory progress. When he talked about his son it was done in such a way that I always felt Oliver was being assessed by a middle-management employment expert with a degree in psychology. His approach was always analytical, punctuated with psychobabble and more suited to the boardroom than that of a caring father describing his son.

At every visit there was a carefully prepared assessment of the progress Oliver had made since the last visit, neatly divided up into the various aspects of his academic life, his general levels of application, and improvements within the home environment and its structure. However, no matter how trivial there was always a downside. Oliver always failed to be perfect in his father's eyes, be it not watching a television program his father thought would be suitable, to only scoring one goal in a soccer match.

Oliver progressed very nicely in spite of his father, though on several occasions I had to sanction his behavior, point out that that is what kids do, and remind his father that Oliver was only eight years old. From start to finish I never once met his mother; with hindsight I suspect that if I had she would have blown the whistle on Oliver's dad's obsessive nature and the strain that this had placed on the marriage. This probably explains why his mother was rarely mentioned and never available apparently to visit the clinic. Apart from giving Oliver's brain a helping hand, I also hope that to some degree I did something toward giving him back his childhood.

The child is certainly father to this man—Brad, aged ten

Brad was brought to see me by his father. His mother had gone off with his father's best friend some eighteen months previously, since when he had lived with his father, with his grandmother filling in until Dad got home from work.

*He had been **born prematurely**, had needed a **forceps-assisted delivery**, had suffered **fetal distress** and was a **poor feeder**, was **late attaining all his developmental milestones** and had displayed signs of developmental delay since being a toddler.*

The examination only served to confirm my suspicions that Brad had a moderately severe form of developmental delay. I provided Brad with some treatment at the clinic and sent them off with a sheaf of papers which covered clearly, item by item, how to change the diet, what to take out and what to add. On a separate sheet was a breakdown of foods to avoid and why, and on yet another sheet a simple step-by-step exercise program.

I arranged to see Brad again in one month's time. Two days later Brad's father rang to cancel the appointment. When I asked why, he said that Brad would not take the supplements, would not eat the food provided, insisted on having sodas and refused to do the exercises. Also, his mother (Brad's grandmother) was too old to put up with all the screaming and had told him she was going to carry on giving Brad his chicken nuggets and oven fries or he could find somebody else to do his baby-sitting.

I suggested we should talk it through, but unfortunately he would not, or could not, bring himself to do that and I never saw the child again.

LITERACY AND DDS

The National Adult Literacy Survey in 1992 showed that 50 percent of Americans age 16 and above have significant problems with reading. Twenty-seven percent of those could not handle reading a newspaper with acceptable comprehension. A follow-up study in 2003 by the same group showed that 14 percent of adults, sixteen and older, had below basic prose literacy. In the 16–18 age group 37 percent of adults had only the most basic reading skills with 11 percent below basic.

This is not only a problem in terms of teaching, but it may also be a further indication of how many children have DDS problems, whether large or small. Testing children and addressing these problems may go a long way to helping solve the huge literacy problem that we have in this country.

If you think you might suffer from some of the symptoms we have described in this book, don't despair, you can also get help. It isn't too late and it will probably change your life for the better.

Adults with DDS will be the subject of my next book as there is a lot of information to give on the subject, partly because it shows itself in different ways in adults than it does in children. What can be said here is that help must be given to children as soon as possible in their lives so that they don't become adults who've slipped through the net.

DDS doesn't go away if untreated—it persists throughout life and causes wider problems once away from the relative protection of school and home.

Here are some strategies for parents who display symptoms:

1. Don't be ashamed to admit you have problems.
2. Seek help yourself.
3. Turn it to your advantage—you can help your child.
4. Grow together—you can both work on the problem together.

What I find in the clinic is that the support of the parents is absolutely key to the treatment of their child. Most of the children are not old enough to take responsibility, and it really is up to the parent to insure that the child follows the program.

Typical reasons given by parents for not sticking with the diet/treatment:

1. We were on vacation.
2. It was the school vacation, so we were out of routine.
3. He was staying away with his father.
4. He has been staying with friends.
5. We just don't have time.
6. He is too busy with schoolwork.
7. The computer crashed.
8. I've been too busy at work.
9. He (a six-year-old) won't do it.

Many other excuses are given, but they all say I want *you* to fix it now as I am too busy with myself.

The following case is a sad one. Reading between the lines, I would hazard a guess that the father also had ADHD symptoms and the mother (it usually is the mother who initiates medical help) tried to do something about making her son better, but because of her own issues she was unable to stick with it.

The ADHD failure—Kevin, aged eleven

Eleven-year-old Kevin was brought to see me by his mother after yet another upset at school, resulting in her being called in to see the principal and the suggestion by him that another school might be better for her son.

When asked about any family history of behavioral or learning disabilities, his mother went to great lengths to explain to me all the problems she had had with his father and all the problems that there were on that side of the family. Needless to say, she denied there were problems on her side, but her overfamiliarity, dogmatism and outright bad manners should have made bells ring right from the start.

The family history, developmental delay, poor diet and examination findings were all textbook in terms of a developmental delay manifesting itself as what we have called ADHD. The treatment should have been straightforward and initially involved no more than changing the diet to exclude bad food additives, artificial sweeteners, the bucketloads of sugar, carbohydrates and fats, while adding omega-3 and omega-6 at double dosage. A simple exercise regime was put in place that would take no more than fifteen minutes a day. Once these dietary changes and the exercise had taken effect and he was more settled and calmer, the second phase of the treatment could be initiated to get the right-prefrontal cortex working the way it was meant to.

At every visit—when visits weren't missed—I would ask about progress and at every visit the mother would provide lame excuses as to why Kevin had not followed my instructions. Off the diet because they were on vacation, not doing the exercises because he had been too busy, off the diet and not doing the exercises because he preferred to play on his Playstation and she, his mother, was too busy to insist that he did.

On the last visit I sat and calmly talked through the problem we were having as I saw it. Clearly the treatment would not, could not work, unless it was undertaken on a regular basis. At this point I was told in no uncertain terms that she was far too busy (in other words, I felt she was really saying that she was far too important) and obviously had to attend to so many things (clothes shopping, meeting friends for coffee, going out to dinner etc.) that she could not be expected to oversee the daily treatment of her son.

She did not make a follow-up appointment but when I rang a month or so later she told me that he had been put on Ritalin®. I wanted to say all the things that were boiling up inside me but thought it best to hold my tongue. I could have told her what I know of the side effects of Ritalin® and the latest research that suggests it may cause long-term brain damage, but she did not want to know that; all she wanted was an immediate solution to the problem so that she could get on with her own life. A short-term solution, yes, but a potentially terrible long-term cost.

Unfortunately, none of us is taught to be parents and, even in cases where there is a problem, little or no support is forthcoming. In fact, unless there are severe problems and the social services step in, parents are left entirely to their own devices when it comes to parenting.

There is no better place or time to learn parenting skills than in the school setting. This would need a courageous step forward at governmental level, but as children are our future it would make good sense, and in the long term save the country billions both in health and education. By teaching the simple skills of parenting in the classroom, there would be instant feedback to the parents and, as the child would be the initiator of change, it would be self-fulfilling providing the parents accepted the teaching.

Whatever the government does or doesn't do in the future, it is clear that parents of DDS children need support and encouragement if their child's treatment is to be successful.

13

ADOLESCENTS AND ADULTS WITH DEVELOPMENTAL DELAY SYNDROME

EARLY DETECTION AND TREATMENT OF DDS

Every parent wants the best for their child and parents of DDS children will probably tend to worry more about their child's future than other parents. In this chapter I will explain how you can give your child the best possible chance in life by detecting and treating developmental delay syndromes so that it does not continue into the teenage years and beyond to adulthood.

What becomes of the child who has an untreated developmental delay as he/she moves into adulthood? Some books on dyslexia, ADHD or other learning disabilities may leave you wondering about the possibilities for your child's future in terms of work and life opportunities. Of course, everyone has free will and some will do what they want to, even with DDS. More usually, without a permanent treatment for the child, their future path may look something like this:

- behavioral difficulties at home and in kindergarten; problems getting on with siblings
- difficulties behaving appropriately at school and getting along with peers
- learning problems, falling behind in class; their self-esteem suffers

- falling behind at school; having trouble passing exams
- difficulty getting accepted into further education
- problems getting and keeping a job
- money problems arising from being unemployed or in low-paid work
- possible trouble with authorities, police
- alcohol and drug problems
- relationship problems

Let's think about the employment prospects of someone whose main symptom was dyslexia in childhood. If the child is not treated and continues to have problems academically this will impact upon examination results as well as the number of examinations they sit. Without a high-school diploma a university education is not possible, and hence career choice is limited. As intellect is not directly related to developmental delay, a possibly very bright person could be stuck in a job that is unfulfilling and less than they'd be capable of without their developmental delay, leaving that person to a lifetime of frustration and relative poverty.

The effects of DDS in adult life (and the possibilities for treatment) are a book in their own right, but here we will look at some of the areas that will impact on the life of the individual as they grow older.

At Tinsley House Clinic we know that, with the right treatment, your child's future can be as rosy as that of an "average" child. The delay that is holding them back can be reduced dramatically or, as with most children we treat, eradicated altogether.

When you become an adult, problems of childhood do not melt away. You do not suddenly develop a brilliant memory, become able to spell, discover you can read or shed the problems you had in childhood. If anything, the situation can only get worse. Some of the problems of childhood will have become a part of your personality—being quiet, a touch obsessive etc.—while others will become a positive hindrance both in your working and social life. Imagine what it must be like trying to get insurance, reading instructions on medicine or planning a vacation if you can't read.

However, it is not all doom and gloom. Many people with DDS have, without treatment, managed to succeed in life, becoming fabulously wealthy, creating breathtaking works of art or expanding the horizons of our knowledge. It is arguable that they succeeded not despite their disability but *because* of it. That is, by having to think outside the box and by not following the dictates of existing thinking, such individuals can approach a situation from a different angle and thereby find a different solution. Perhaps this is what we call lateral thinking.

For parents of children who have childhood symptoms of ADHD, things get much harder in adolescence if it is left untreated. ADHD is often followed by oppositional defiance disorder. That is, the hyperactivity and behavioral problems of the ADHD child can worsen, and blatant defiance and direct confrontation can ensue. As the child gets physically bigger and the sex hormones kick in, the situation can get completely out of hand with physical violence and antisocial behavior bringing the youth into direct confrontation with the law. Alcohol and drug abuse can cause the sufferer to spiral out of control, leading to mindless acts of vandalism and unprovoked acts of extreme violence. This is a depressing downhill path, leaving the parents wondering just what they did wrong. The prospects for the sufferer of being in and out of work, and possibly having a string of failed relationships, are not comforting.

When I speak of treatment for ADHD, I don't mean using drugs. The prescribed drugs used to treat ADHD are not actually a treatment at all, as it would appear that Ritalin® only suppresses the aspects of ADHD, making the child better behaved and manageable, but does not actually treat the underlying cause of the disorder. Not only does Ritalin® fail to treat the condition; new evidence suggests that it actually causes long-term brain damage—for a relatively short period of time the drug masks the symptoms but, in so doing, is said to damage the brain permanently. When you consider that it is not just children with ADHD that are taking this drug, but completely asymptomatic children, who are using it illegally as an academic performance enhancer, the prospects for the future of our children becomes frightening.

Obsessive-compulsive disorder of childhood can progress into a far more worrying adult form, but more commonly becomes built into the sufferer's personality. In its mildest form this may manifest itself as an overwhelming desire to keep cupboards and drawers overly tidy with almost military precision—tins organized by size and content and all facing forward and positioned to within a millimeter.

At the extreme, this personality type may be impossible to live with, as no one can live in an environment that has to be perfect 24 hours a day. It can generate unbearable stress, lead to marital breakdown and place the children of this kind of parent in a highly charged emotional situation from which they cannot escape.

In childhood the signs of Tourette's syndrome can be so subtle that even parents don't notice them until they are pointed out. In fact it is likely that these minor signs of Tourette's and the other symptoms of developmental delay may be normal glitches in the early development of the brain. In childhood the inner desire to give in to the urge to tic or grimace can make the child feel guilty or ashamed and add to the stress a lot of children face in trying to live up to their parents' expectations and their peers' achievements. In adulthood, having Tourette's can lead to a person living a restricted lifestyle where they avoid certain situations. Often they not only suffer from the inner turmoil this condition produces but also the humiliating responses they get from people who don't understand the affliction.

We have looked at the impact untreated dyslexia can have in the long term, disadvantaging the sufferer both in terms of achieving their potential in life and in gaining the financial reward such success might bring. However, the other symptoms of developmental delay can also impact upon our lives, both in directing the paths we take in life and in coloring what we call our personality. Obsessive behavior can be the cause of a great deal of family tension but obsessive attention to detail can be of great benefit to an employer. Similarly, the individual with Asperger's can drive you to despair while you are trying to unwind on a relaxing weekend away, yet, as an advisor, that same person could be a godsend if he or she happened to be handling your financial affairs.

Some smart employers know this and it does not take too long for the psychology graduate in the personnel department to put our little foibles to good use.

SOME FAMOUS PEOPLE KNOWN TO HAVE DEVELOPMENTAL DELAY

Actors: Tom Cruise, Whoopi Goldberg, Dustin Hoffman, Steve McQueen, Sylvester Stallone, Robin Williams, Anthony Hopkins

Leaders: Dwight Eisenhower, Napoleon Bonaparte, George Patton, Winston Churchill, Benjamin Franklin, Woodrow Wilson, Nelson Rockefeller, John F. Kennedy

Writers and artists: William Butler Yeats, Agatha Christie, Hans Christian Andersen, Edgar Allan Poe, Jules Verne, Rodin, Leonardo da Vinci, Gustave Flaubert, Charles Schulz

Musicians: Cher, Harry Belafonte, Ludwig van Beethoven, Wolfgang Amadeus Mozart, John Lennon

Scientists: Thomas Edison, Michael Faraday, Albert Einstein, Alexander Graham Bell, Galileo, Stephen Hawking, Louis Pasteur, Charles Darwin, Harvey Cushing (US neurologist)

Entrepreneurs: Henry Ford, Bill Gates, Howard Hughes

SUCCESSFUL PEOPLE WITH DDS—AN EXAMPLE

I was recently asked if I could cover for a colleague and provide a series of lectures in the very beautiful European city of Bologna. On the first morning of the lectures I was pleasantly surprised to notice that an old colleague of mine from the days when I was training had entered the room. I had always admired Bernard's intellect and was therefore very pleased to see my old friend and have the opportunity for some long conversations.

Normally, in the lecture room Bernard remains silent, soaking up whatever is being offered to him, but this weekend was to be different. Throughout the weekend he questioned me and, much to the amusement of the rest of the audience, a great deal of intellectual fencing went on. At first I had thought that Bernard was questioning me because he had the mental prowess to do just that, but I quickly came to realize that the theories I had proposed had obviously appealed greatly to Bernard. He was merely checking out various aspects of my theories, as if he were to consider accepting my various proposals he would have to reorganize much of his past learning. It was this very reorganization that was fundamental to his precise analytical approach to everything I was saying.

In the past I had teased Bernard about his OCD traits but I had not realized just how structured this brilliant mind had to be. In order to accept this new information, huge areas of his past learning would have to be restructured so that there would always be a continuum.

Over the weekend I turned Bernard's learning line (not a learning curve) into a game and would tease him, kindly, each time he needed a further explanation. I had noticed that every time he mentioned a book, as in, "Have you read Goldberg?" it would be followed by a comment such as, "That is the black book with yellow writing."

Therefore, often my answer would be, "Yes, but have you read Bradshaw, that is the blue book with the black writing?" However, as the weekend progressed, I noticed how closely our thinking processes were mirrored by each other and how aspects of OCD and Asperger's can drive a focused mind to new realms of understanding.

If the child's main problem is dyslexia the obvious immediate effect will be falling behind at school. As dyslexia never occurs in isolation, aspects of dyspraxia associated with it may make the clumsy child the subject of ridicule or bullying. We all know children say what they see and can therefore appear to be very cruel. The hidden impact of this on the child can range from low self-esteem to anxiety or depression. As the right side of the brain is the "approach/withdrawal" decision maker and under-functions in 98 percent of children with problems, children with developmental delay see danger everywhere. They are therefore fragile individuals in the first place and this is easily dented by bad school reports, remarks from unthinking parents or teachers, and teasing and/or bullying by other children. This in itself is a tragedy of childhood but we must bear in mind that this damaged fragile personality will be carried over into adult life and will have an impact throughout that individual's life.

Untreated, the child with dyslexic problems will not only fall behind but stay behind in their schooling, which of course will impact upon their exam results and ultimately influence their possible choices of career. Therefore, the child who could have grown up to be a successful attorney ends up misplaced in society, perhaps never achieving their potential.

The following case study shows how all the things we have talked about so far can impact on the child and potentially destroy their future.

Dan, aged fourteen

At fourteen Dan had already fallen behind at school, been moved from one school to another and, because his parents could afford it, was sent to boarding school. In reality Dan was a frightened child who needed constant reassurance, love and support—he needed to be within a strong, functional family. As it was, his parents were divorced, were constantly criticizing one another and gave gifts or money in place of love.

Kids that struggle emotionally and educationally often adopt strategies for coping. This can involve acting the fool, as this—at least initially—bonds you with your classmates. When Dan could not cope in class he would do anything to get a laugh, or be defiant or rude to the teaching staff to demonstrate to his friends how tough he was. This had led to him being in trouble on numerous occasions and eventually to him being suspended.

However, when the school contacted his mother she was not initially interested and, when told she had to remove him from the school, took him out for the day for a feast of junk food and shopping for still more unnecessary gifts. Dan's long-practiced skills in bending the truth had his mother believing his innocence within minutes. By accepting his version of the events leading up to his suspension, she freed herself of any responsibility and could get on with her life, which was why Dan was at boarding school in the first place.

By constantly ignoring Dan's cries for help she was pushing him further and further into the depths of despair, and now his outbursts in class were no longer considered amusing by his peers. Somehow he had to at least regain respect from his peers and in an attempt to do this he took up smoking. He now distanced himself from his mother, referring to her as "that cow" and on the rare occasions that he went home for the weekend would be both verbally and physically aggressive toward her.

Back at school the cigarettes, to which he was rapidly becoming addicted, were not having the effect he had hoped for with his peers, and so he had started drinking heavily whenever the opportunity arose and he had negotiated with another older pupil to buy drugs. His plan was simple. Alone as he was, without friends now inside or outside school, he would cultivate a little business that would earn him good money and the money would make him feel good. Unfortunately, in order to buy the drugs he had to associate with some very unsavoury characters and, within the school, develop a network of other struggling pupils in order to let the pupils at large know he was selling.

It was when his master plan fell apart that eventually his mother brought him to me for treatment and I found signs of developmental delay and its impact on his life. Unfortunately, when his mother discovered that she could not just leave him with me to fix, she decided not to continue with treatment. Instead she moved him to yet another new school that would accept him and got on with her life.

Unfortunately, I don't know what has become of Dan.

There is always hope—Millie, aged four

*Millie's mother contacted the clinic initially by e-mail, providing a long and detailed history of Millie's developmental history, or rather lack of it. She had been born at full-term following a painfully long labor but was delivered naturally without assistance and had breast-fed without difficulty. However, she had **failed to thrive mentally or physically** to the point that she had been seen locally and at a well-known London hospital, but without the all-important diagnosis that every parent in this situation wants and yet dreads. Even genetic testing had drawn a blank.*

*When seen at the clinic three weeks later four-year-old Millie was **in a world of her own**, and even when she had become familiar with her new surroundings, she made **limited eye contact** and **refused to speak** or cooperate. In this situation all you can do is observe and* *wait until you find a chink in the armor. By this time Millie was on the floor and I had joined her and, more by luck than judgement, I happened to look into a carrier bag that was next to her mother. Fortunately, both Millie and I had had a misspent childhood and the sight of sausage rolls was just too much for me. Once the sausage rolls were in my hands Millie suddenly became very attentive and exceedingly cooperative.*

*Not wishing to push my luck, even from my position of strength, I conducted all the tests I needed to be sure and safe that I knew what I was dealing with and left it at that. My guess was that Millie had suffered, unnoticed, from **fetal distress**, she was not brain-damaged as such but her brain was struggling to cope, let alone develop. Remembering the words of my wise professor I decided to do very little in terms of treatment and observe the results.*

Her treatment program included:

1. *the Tinsley Clinic Diet*
2. *supplements*
3. *cerebellar exercises*
4. *using subtle shock tactics to stimulate the brain stem*
5. *computer-generated programs to stimulate set areas of the brain*

This proved to be the right choice and over a period of weeks Millie began to change. She appeared to be more aware of her environment, able to communicate her needs and was no longer locked away in her own little world. It would be months before Millie would be able to function independently, but each day when she snuggled up to her mother, something she had never done before, little else seemed to matter and she has time on her side.

A LETTER FROM A "DYSLEXIC" ADULT

The alarm goes off, that familiar feeling of dread floods my body as I know it's that time again, yes, school. A place that for some can mean looking forward to the new novel that's being given out in the next English lesson, or perhaps it would be learning the lines for a favored part in the play, but for others it can simply mean how can I get through today without people sniggering at me when I can't read a sentence out loud let alone a page properly in English or only having half the notes written down from lessons because you can't keep up with the dictation. The continual thought that something was not quite right and with no one to recognize there was a problem with my ability to learn to read etc., understand new topics or generally fit in with the rest of my peers.

My way of dealing with this unfortunate situation was to act as if I didn't care and entertain classmates with trying to be the comedian in a flippant jovial manner that although it may have come across as though I really had no interest at all in any of the subjects being taught, really it was a release of pent-up frustration of not knowing why I couldn't do what seemed so natural to the other children and learn!

I write these words now as a 30 year old reflecting on my school years and also my life up until three years ago, when on a rare occasion I attempted to read the paper, I quite literally stumbled across an article on dyslexia which struck a chord deep within me that even if I had attained a brilliant degree in English at university, I would still struggle to describe! I wasn't alone, perhaps I might not be that thick and maybe there might even be some help out there.

Doing invariably unskilled manual labor until relatively recently even the simplest tasks seemed to strike an air of confusion, from navigating lanes on roundabouts, writing an order for egg and fries when working in a café with the eager customer peering at the order sheet with a look of disdain as I write "eggs on flies!" to helping my niece read one of her story books when she was only eight and she actually read it better than me (she is a very bright little girl I must add!).

However, on a more positive note and taking advantage of different therapies ranging from listening to Mozart, with a view to gain right-ear dominance, looking through a Syntonizer at different lights for an hour a day for two weeks to open the fields of vision, to being caught by my housemates walking up the stairs with my eyes shut and holding a tray with a glass of water on it to help stimulate the left cerebellum! I have made significant and continual progress to enjoy life and a career of which I thought I would never have and was once destined not to.

To conclude, I could look back on my earlier years with a degree of pity and perhaps a justified degree of blame maybe even anger that I wasn't helped at an earlier age, but that really isn't going to help and would probably serve to my detriment as no one can live with blame and regrets in their lives and be truly happy. All I hope is that as the understanding of dyslexia increases so the treatments and therapies improve and others in a similar position can get the help needed.

I like to think of my earlier years to my advantage, as every ounce of progress I make now, whether it be reading a chapter of a novel with fluid understanding or laughing at a joke that once made no sense but now makes me laugh, is that much sweeter.

Sure, perhaps if there was such a thing as a magic cure when I was younger maybe I could have been an astronaut. But there is still plenty of time and the stars are still shining bright!

GC

OTHER ISSUES FOR ADULT SUFFERERS

The understanding of learning and behavioral difficulties as conditions in their own right, and the discovery of developmental delay, is so new that we cannot say with certainty what the results in adulthood will be if it is untreated.

The implications of untreated developmental delay could extend into a range of potentially very dangerous behavioral problems that may include such things as road rage and truly psychopathic behavior. An imbalance between the controling centers in the prefrontal cortex and the primitive centers at the base of the brain might well explain why the physical signs of increased heart rate, raised blood pressure and unrestrained anger lead sufferers of road rage, for instance, to have an inability to let things pass and the overriding need to settle the score, no matter what the cost or how trivial the event.

Under normal circumstances, if you have to run for a bus you do not want to unleash the full "fight or flight" response and we therefore use a short-term strategy called the "vagal brake." By doing this we can take the blood pressure up, increase the heart rate and increase the respiratory rate and hopefully catch the bus without feeling the after-effects of a massive adrenaline rush. Some people, however, do not seem to be able to do this and so operate on an all-or-nothing basis throughout life.

Being able to interpret body language or non-verbal communication such as gestures or facial expressions is the job of the prefrontal cortex and needs those special brain cells that develop four months after birth. We also know that this same area is vital in the control of our most basic urges. At this stage we can only speculate but it would seem likely that extreme, violent behavior is a product of an underdeveloped prefrontal cortex, and that the lack of remorse following a brutal act against another person or animal would also indicate a total inability to know right from wrong, which again would be a function of this same area of brain.

Research carried out in America, the UK and Spain has shown that a chemical involved in the functioning of neurotransmitters in the brain is normally very high in young people, notably boys, but thankfully this usually declines as we get older. It has been suggested that it is the high level of this chemical in the brains of youths that accounts for their inability to see danger. Abnormally high levels of this chemical have been found to be present in adults who indulge in dangerous sports and also in criminals who have committed savage crimes for which they feel no remorse whatsoever.

This area of research is so new that we must wait until researchers around the globe pick up on various aspects of it before we see clear evidence of the extent of just what these new brain cells do, and the impact this might have on our development. It may also open up new avenues of research into the genetic control of brain development and, if looked at from this new perspective, it may cause researchers to take a fresh look at a range of disorders that afflict us. It is also worth mentioning that, while research suggests there are connections between them, it doesn't by any means mean that a child with learning disabilities will develop any or all of the following.

Schizophrenia

The root cause of schizophrenia may lie in the delayed or abnormal development of the same brain cells that are involved in the generation of developmental delay. Indeed current research is looking closely at the neurotransmitter dopamine. There are two principal centers in the brain stem that produce large quantities of dopamine. The first area produces dopamine for the basal nuclei and when this production of dopamine starts to fail, Parkinson's disease starts to develop. The second area of dopamine production provides dopamine for the prefrontal cortex, the very area of brain we have been considering throughout this book, and it may well be that a "chicken and egg" situation occurs between these two areas. If the second area of dopamine production is under-functioning it will have an impact on the prefrontal cortex and vice versa. Interestingly, another area of research has looked at the early development of people who went on to suffer from schizophrenia. Not surprisingly, many of these patients had shown signs during childhood that were considered autistic or fell in line with what we now know to be developmental delay.

Dementia and Alzheimer's

It is of interest to note that the second wave of brain cells that are involved in the generation of the symptoms of developmental delay are also the earliest cells to suffer in the onset of dementia and Alzheimer's disease. We know that the outcome in terms of recovery from a stroke, for instance, depends upon where it happens and how bad it is, but also upon how fit the brain was before the stroke occurred.

Similarly, we know that the outward signs of dementia will vary depending on just how fit the brain was before the onset. That is, if you had two people, one of whom was a "mental athlete," exercising her brain on a daily basis—doing crossword puzzles or reading avidly—while the other was a mental couch potato, and they both suffered exactly the same degree of dementia, the mental athlete would outwardly have far less signs of dementia. This is, of course, exactly the same situation you would expect with muscle loss. If you and the strongest man in the world lost half of your physical strength, the strongest man would still be much stronger than you.

There is no research to prove it but logic would dictate that if these brain cells that are likely to be the first to suffer with the onset of Alzheimer's were not functioning as they should from childhood onwards, then the effects of the dementia is likely to be much greater than if they were fully fit and functional. It has been suggested that with our modern diet of pre-prepared processed convenience foods we should all be taking omega-3 and omega-6 on a daily basis, and early evidence would suggest that this might in fact delay or even prevent the onset of dementia.

CONCLUSION

The discovery that the human brain has a second wave of brain cells that develop when the child is at four months of age really was an amazing breakthrough. It was this realization that led to the Tinsley House Clinic treatment.

The aim of *The Learning Disability Myth* is to help you to identify your child's problem effectively and then to get a proper diagnosis; to take some steps toward feeding them a diet that will support their brain and enable it to mature and function as it should. At the end of the process I want you to be able to say, "This is my child: a child who is healthier, happier, coping better at school and who has a higher level of self-esteem."

As we learn more about the brain and how it works, we can identify the location of the problems and can now offer treatments that are lasting and effective. At Tinsley House Clinic we believe that this is just the beginning of all that is possible with the human brain.

It may feel like the end of the world when your child is diagnosed with a learning or behavioral difficulty, but it really is not all doom and gloom. The most exciting part of the work that we do at Tinsley House is seeing the results we achieve and the very real improvements we make to children's lives.

It will take a little time and effort to make changes in your child's life where diet is concerned but it will make all the difference to the functioning of their brain as well as to their future health and longevity.

We know that your child can be treated and has the ability to fulfill their potential and go on to lead a "normal" life and the best life they can. What more can any parent ask for their child?

GLOSSARY

Accommodation/convergence failure—The inability of the eyes to move in toward the nose when looking at something close up, e.g. when reading

Acetylcholine—a substance used by nerves to send messages to other nerves

Afferentating—causing messages to be sent into the nervous system

Arachidonic acid—a polyunsaturated fatty acid that is essential for growth

Archiocortex—the outer layer of the brain is called the cortex: there are three types of cortex—archio, paleo and neocortex—the first two are called the primitive cortex (older) while the last type is the newest in terms of brain evolution

Asperger's syndrome—a disorder in which the individual shows marked deficiencies in social skills, does not like change, often has obsessive routines and becomes preoccupied with particular subjects

Attention deficit disorder (ADD)—an inability to focus/concentrate on the job in hand, with a tendency to be easily distracted—tends to go hand in hand with ADHD—it is a classic symptom of developmental delay

Attention deficit hyperactivity disorder (ADHD)—as for ADD above but with aspects of hyperactivity and impulsivity

Autism (true)—affects about 1 in 5000 children, being four times more common in boys than girls—it has been thought for some time to be due to abnormal brain development and now would appear to be due to a lack of spindle cells—autistic children avoid eye contact, shun affection, do not understand other people's emotions/feelings, have problems making friends and cannot adjust to the rules of society

Autistic spectrum disorder (ASD)—affects 9 in 1000 children— these children display autistic tendencies, and it may well prove to be an extreme form of developmental delay due to reduced numbers of spindle cells or greatly impaired spindle cell development

Azo dye—a synthetic dye, usually red, brown or yellow, that makes up about half the food dyes we use

Benzoate—chemical used as a food preserver

Brain stem—the part of the nervous system that joins the brain to the spinal cord: it contains many of the vital centers—vital because without them you die

Carcinogen—a substance thought to cause cancer

Cerebellar hemisphere—the cerebellum has a middle section with a large lobe on either side called a hemisphere

Cerebellum—literally "little brain" that lives in the very back of the skull under the brain

Cerebral hemisphere—the name given to either side of the brain

Choline—a dietary component of many foods—forms part of many major phospholipids

Chromosomal—to do with chromosomes, which are the thread-like structures found in the nucleus cells and which carry the genes

Congenital—present at birth

Cranial nerves—twelve pairs of nerves found at the base of the brain and brain stem

Cross-cord reflexes—messages that get passed from one side of the spinal cord to the other so that we can do things like walking, swimming etc.

Diaschisis—put simply this is when one area of the brain does not work too well because an area it normally communicates with has a problem (it's a bit like a couple having a row and not talking to each other)

Docosahexaenoic acid—an omega-3 essential fatty acid

Dopamine signaling—messages sent from one nerve to another using a special substance—a neurotransmitter—called dopamine

Dressing dyspraxia—difficulty dressing

Dysarthria—inability to produce clear speech

Dysdiadochokinesia—the inability to make rapidly alternating movements—turning the hands/palm up and down

Dyslexia—a term used to cover a variety of learning disabilities

Dysmetria—inaccurate movements

Dyspraxia—an inability to perform learned movements accurately—can take many forms and has been found to be present in association with the other symptoms of developmental delay in over 90 percent of children

Echolalia—repeating what you have just heard

Eicosapentaenoic acid—an omega-3 essential fatty acid

Fat emulsifier—a substance that helps to keep together substances that normally would not go together—e.g. oil and water

Fetal distress—when the fetal heartbeat rises or drops dramatically

Functional dominance—when one area of the brain is superior or dominant in function

Gamma-linoleic acid—an omega-6 essential fatty acid

Humectant—a substance that attracts water and therefore helps to keep a food substance moist

Hygroscopic—readily absorbs water

Inositol—a food substance found notably in cereals

Interneurons—small nerves that interconnect with other nerves

Lecithin—a fatlike substance called a phospholipid which is a fat emulsifier

Linoleic acid—an omega-6 essential fatty acid

Linolenic acid—an omega-6 essential fatty acid

Meconium—the first stool a baby passes

Motor planning—how the brain plans what it is it wants to do

Motor skills—the ability to carry out physical things you have learned to do

Myelin—the fatty insulation that covers nerve fibers

Myelination—the process that takes place during development when certain nerves are wrapped in myelin

Myopic—being nearsighted

Neocortex—in terms of evolution, the newest parts of the brain

Neuroanatomy—the anatomy of the nervous system

Neurologist—an expert in neurology

Neurology—the study of the nervous system

Neurons—nerves

Neurotransmitter—a chemical substance that passes messages from one nerve to the next

Nystagmus—the flickering of the eyes from side to side

Obsessive-compulsive disorder (OCD)—is characterized by a recurrent urge to carry out ritualistic behavior patterns—it is a common symptom of developmental delay—to a certain extent we all have minor aspects of compulsive behavior, only becoming a problem when it occurs to such a degree that it takes over a person's waking life

Oppositional defiance disorder (ODD)—European description: conduct seen in children below ten years of age characterized by markedly defiant, disobedient or provocative behavior. American description: a pattern of hostile, negative, defiant behavior lasting at least six months during which four of the following occur: often loses temper, often argues with adults, often actively defies or refuses to comply with requests/rules, often deliberately annoys others, often blames others for his/her mistakes, is easily annoyed, is often angry, is often spiteful

Otoacoustic emission tests—a hearing test of inner-ear function

Otoscope—the device used by doctors for looking in the ear

Paliocortex—one of the more primitive (older) types of the outer layer of the brain (cortex)

Peripheral nerves—nerves that leave the brain/brain stem/spinal cord

Peripheral nervous system (PNS)—the nervous system is divided in the central nervous system (brain/brain stem/spinal cord) and the peripheral nervous system (all the nerves that leave or enter the central nervous system)

Phosphatidyl serine—a component of the cell membrane called phospholipids

Phosphoglyceride—a type of phospholipids

Phospholipids—a fatty component of the cell wall

Prefrontal cortex—a large area of brain (in humans) at the front of the brain

Prosody—the musical quality of language, as opposed to a flat monotone

Prostaglandins—a member of a group of fats made from omega-3 and omega-6

Sequestrant—a food additive that binds with metals, which might have got into the food by accident, thus making them inert

Spindle cells—special brain cells (nerves) that develop four months after birth in humans—they are only found in the brains of the great apes and Man—it is considered that these cells and the development of the prefrontal cortex (the front of the brain) is what makes us truly human

Temporal sequencing—fitting events into a time frame

Titubation—rocking to and fro

Tourette's syndrome—generally considered to be a condition in which a tic (involuntary movement) is associated with the sufferer swearing uncontrollably—however, minor aspects of it appear in so many children in the form of excessive blinking, grimacing or throat clearing for it to be considered a normal aspect of development

Tympanometry test—a special hearing test that assesses how well the eardrum and middle ear is functioning

Vagal brake—one way in which the brain controls the heart rate, blood pressure and respiration rate

Ventouse—an assisted birth using suction to pull the baby through the birth canal

RECIPES

(drawn up by Jacqueline Burns)

Pancakes with banana and honey filling

125g (4.5oz) plain flour
1 egg
1 cup milk
oil for frying
banana, sliced
honey

(Batter needs to be made an hour before using.)

1   Measure the flour into a bowl. Make a well in the center, add the egg and pour in a little of the milk.
2   Using a wooden spoon or an electric mixer beat until smooth, adding the rest of the milk slowly.
3   Put the mixture aside for at least an hour.
4   Using a tablespoon of oil, heat the frying pan until it is extremely hot, just before it starts to smoke. (You will need to add more oil before each pancake is cooked.)
5   Pour the batter into a jug for easy pouring, or use a ladle. Pour in enough batter to thinly cover the bottom of the pan and tilt the pan to spread evenly.
6   You can lift with an egg slice, at the sides to see if it is cooked

underneath; it will be a little golden. Don't flip over until the underneath is done.

7   Lift out of the pan, put the sliced banana along one side of the pancake, drizzle with a little honey and roll or fold up.

Houmous wraps

pitta bread
houmous
any crunchy strips of vegetables that your child will eat, such as red
    pepper, tomato, cucumber or carrot (uncooked)

1   Generously spread the pitta bread with houmous.
2   Add some of the vegetable crunchy strips.
3   Roll up and wrap in foil or greaseproof paper.

Spaghetti and Meatballs

This will make plenty for the whole family for dinner and have leftovers for lunch.

500g (17.5oz) ground pork
500g (17.5oz) ground beef
1 medium onion, finely chopped
2 tablespoons of parsley, finely chopped
1 can of tomatoes
olive oil for frying
wholemeal spaghetti (this may take some adjustment for your child
    but will be worth it)
1 cupful of grated Parmesan

1   Combine the ground pork and beef, onion and parsley in a bowl and mix well.
2   Then shape the meatballs into round balls about the size of a 50 cent piece.
3   Heat a tablespoon of olive oil in the pan and fry the meatballs until browned evenly.
4   Empty the can of tomatoes into the pan, including juice, and

cook for about 20 minutes until the sauce separates from the meatballs.

5 Meanwhile, cook enough spaghetti for your child, to the specifications on the packet.

6 Serve with grated parmesan on top of the meatballs.

Home-made mini-burgers
This can also be used for lunches.

500g (17.5oz) ground beef
½ apple, peeled and grated
1 sweet potato, cooked and mashed
½ onion, finely chopped
1 egg
olive oil for frying

1 Combine all ingredients—except the olive oil—in a bowl.

2 Shape into burgers to a size to suit your child's appetite.

3 Heat oil in a frying pan and fry each burger for 5–10 minutes on each side until browned (flatter burgers will cook more quickly).

4 The rest of the mixture—shaped into larger burgers—can be used for an adult meal.

Home-made fries

potatoes suitable for frying (it will say on the bag if they are suitable), cut into French fries
olive oil

1 Place a baking pan with 3 tablespoons of oil into the oven for 10 minutes on 400°F (gas mark 6).

2 When the pan is heated, place the fries into the pan and toss in the oil until they are evenly coated.

3 Cook for 20 minutes (or more, depending on the thickness of your fries). Check and move in the oil every 5 minutes or so. When they are soft, and crispy on the outside, they are done.

Oven-roasted chicken drumsticks

chicken drumsticks (most supermarkets do reasonably cheap large packs)
olive oil

1 Place drumsticks in a roasting pan and drizzle with olive oil.
2 Roast for 20 minutes on 350°F (gas mark 4), checking and basting every 5 minutes or so.
3 They are cooked when you insert a sharp knife near the bone and the juices run clear.

These drumsticks can be served with broccoli, sweetcorn or carrots. Or if your child loves potatoes, cut some into 2cm cubes and roast along with the chicken.

Chilli con carne and rice with grated cheese

500g (17.5oz) ground beef
1 can of red kidney beans
1 can of tomatoes
1 red pepper, cut into strips
1 large onion, chopped
2 cloves of garlic, crushed
2 tablespoons of olive oil
grated cheese
rice, to taste (brown rice is better for your children but will take
    longer to cook)

1 Heat oil in a large saucepan, add onion and garlic and fry for 5 minutes until soft.
2 Add beef and fry until it loses its pink color.
3 Stir in red pepper, kidney beans and tomatoes (including their sauce), cover with a lid and simmer for an hour.
4 Meanwhile, cook enough rice for your child, to the specifications on the packet.
5 Serve with the rice and grated cheese on top.
6 You can always make enough for the adults too, and add one or two teaspoons of chilli powder in for you to eat.

Spaghetti Bolognese

500g (17.5oz) ground beef
1 cup beef stock (use a stock cube in water)
1 can of tomatoes
3 tablespoons of tomato purée
1 onion, finely chopped
1 clove of garlic, finely chopped
1 carrot, chopped
1 celery stalk, chopped
125g (4.5oz) mushrooms, sliced
25g (1oz) butter, cut into small pieces
1 tablespoon of olive oil
wholemeal spaghetti, to taste (this may take some adjustment for your child but will be worth it)

1   Heat the oil in a saucepan.
2   Fry the onion, garlic, carrot and celery for about 10 minutes until softened.
3   Add the ground beef until browned and then add all other ingredients except the butter and spaghetti. Simmer for 30 minutes.
4   Cook the spaghetti for 10–12 minutes (or to the specifications on the packet), drain and toss in the butter.
5   Pour the sauce over the spaghetti and serve.

If your child is older and you feel happy doing so, you can also add ½ cup red wine in stage 3. The alcohol will burn off but will leave a richer flavor.

Fisher girl/boy's pie

450g (16oz) cod fillet
200g (7oz) smoked haddock fillet
6 large shrimp or a handful of smaller shrimp, cooked
1kg (2½lb) potatoes
1 small onion, sliced
2 cups milk
1 cup double cream

4 eggs

100g (3.5oz) butter

45g (1.5oz) plain flour

4 tablespoons flat-leaf parsley, chopped

1   Preheat the oven to 400°F (gas mark 6).

2   Boil the potatoes until tender. Drain and mash, using ½ cup of the milk to make a soft mash.

3   Set the eggs to boil for 8 minutes. When cool, peel them and slice.

4   Put the onion slices, 1½ cups of the milk, all the cream and both pieces of fish into a large pan. Bring gently to the boil and simmer for 8 minutes.

5   Remove the fish, flake it and spread over the bottom of a large oven dish with the shrimp.

6   Strain the liquid into a jug.

7   Place the boiled egg slices over the fish.

8   Melt 50g (1.75oz) of the butter in a saucepan, add the flour and stir for 1 minute. Remove from the heat and stir in the liquid from the fish.

9   Return to the heat and gently bring to the boil, stirring constantly. Simmer for 10 minutes.

10 Take off the heat, stir in the parsley and pour the sauce over the fish. Leave to cool for half an hour.

11 Spread the mashed potato over the mixture and make lines on the top with the back of a fork.

12 Bake for 30–40 minutes until the potato is a golden-brown color.

Hidden vegetable pasta sauce

This recipe will feed the whole family. If you're using only for your child or children, there'll be some left over to freeze for another meal.

2 carrots, chopped

1 stick of celery, chopped

1 large onion, chopped

1 clove of garlic, chopped

2 sprigs of parsley, chopped

2 cans of tomatoes
pinch of sugar
1 tablespoon of butter
1 tablespoon of olive oil

1   Put the vegetables and tomatoes in a large saucepan. Add the sugar, butter and olive oil.
2   Bring to the boil, turn down the heat immediately and simmer gently for an hour.
3   Put through a mouli or push through a sieve with a back of a spoon. (Don't use a food processor or it will turn to tomato juice consistency.)

Tacos with chicken

Serves 4. Use as much or as little of each ingredient as you like; this recipe is about giving the child choice.

4 taco shells
3 or 4 chicken breasts with skin (depending on how much you eat)
lettuce, shredded
Cheddar cheese, grated
avocado, peeled and sliced
tomatoes, finely diced
red peppers, diced or sliced
olive oil for frying

1   Place chicken breasts skin-side down in a frying pan for about 6 minutes.
2   Place them in an oven-proof dish and put in the oven at 400°F (gas mark 6) for 10 minutes.
3   Once cooked, slice up the chicken into bite-sized pieces and put into a bowl.
4   Make small bowls of the other healthy ingredients that your child can choose from including: lettuce, tomatoes, red peppers, cheddar cheese and avocado.
5   Heat taco shells to the specifications on the packet.
6   Let your child fill the shells with chicken and each of the other ingredients to their liking.

(If you have the time you could make guacamole with the avocado by mashing it up and adding some of the tomato, some finely chopped garlic if your children like it, a dash of lemon juice, and, if you like, a small pinch of salt and pepper.)

Parmesan carrots

Carrots, chopped (the amount should depend on the taste of your family)
Parmesan, grated (enough to sprinkle on the carrots)
1 tsp butter
honey (optional)

1   Steam or boil the carrots until they are cooked and drain the water off.
2   Keeping them in the hot pan, add the butter and Parmesan.
3   Add a touch of honey if your child likes it.

This recipe can also be made with peas instead of carrots, in which case I would recommend tiny pieces of chopped ham instead of the honey.

Fish cakes

450g (1 1b) floury potatoes, chopped
450g (1 1b) firm white fish fillets (such as cod, haddock)
1 egg, beaten
70g (2.5oz) fresh breadcrumbs
25g (1oz) plain flour
15g (0.5oz) butter, melted
1 tablespoon of flat-leaf parsley, chopped
sunflower oil for frying

1   Boil potatoes until tender. Drain and mash. Leave to cool.
2   Bring to the boil in a large deep frying pan enough water to cover the fish. Put in the fish and simmer for 10 minutes.
3   Remove the fish. Once it is cool, break it into flakes.

4   Put the mashed potato and fish into a bowl. Add the melted butter and parsley and mix. (You can also add 1 cup of the bread-crumbs to the mix, if you wish.)

5   Shape into round fishcakes of about 2.5cm thick. Place the fish-cakes on a plate, cover and put in the fridge for 20 minutes.

6   Heat enough oil for deep-frying.

7   Put the flour, beaten egg and breadcrumbs in three separate bowls. Dip the refrigerated fishcakes first in the flour, then the egg and then breadcrumbs.

8   Deep-fry a few at a time for about 4 minutes until golden brown. Place on kitchen paper to absorb oil and then serve.

Pasta with cream, onion and peas

pasta, to taste (white or wholemeal)
1 knob butter
2 shallots (or ½ onion), finely chopped
1 clove garlic, finely chopped
1 big slice ham, finely chopped
½ cup double cream
1 big handful peas (these can be fresh or frozen)
a few tablespoons of Parmesan, grated
salt and pepper to taste

1   Melt the butter in a saucepan, then gently sweat the onion for 5–10 minutes until soft.

2   Add the garlic and ham and fry for a minute or two.

3   Reduce heat to very low (put a diffuser under the pan if you have one), pour in the cream and add the peas. Cook for five minutes.

4   Stir in a tablespoon or two of Parmesan and the pepper (making sure it's finely ground, so your child can't see it).

5   Meanwhile, cook your pasta, according to the specifications on the packet, and add it to the saucepan. Stir to coat the pasta evenly and serve with more Parmesan on top.

If your child is older and you feel happy doing so, you can add ½ glass dry white wine after you've fried the garlic and ham. Boil on a high heat until almost all the liquid has reduced away, then continue the recipe at stage 3.

Chicken liver pâté

This is enough for sandwiches for lunch and breakfast toast for 2 adults and 2 children.

½kg chicken livers
190g butter
2 onions, chopped
3 large mushrooms, chopped
½ green pepper, chopped
1 garlic clove, chopped

1   Melt about half the butter in a large pan. Fry the garlic and onions gently until soft and transparent.
2   Add the chicken livers and fry until they start to brown, which will take about 3 minutes.
3   Add the pepper and mushrooms and fry gently for another 3 minutes.
4   Blend the mixture in a food processor until smooth.
5   Melt the other half of the butter and pour into the blended mixture, stirring in well.
6   Spoon the mixture into a loaf-shaped cake pan or a ceramic pot. (It can go into any container really but either of these make it look better, and an oblong or rectangular one will make it easier to slice.)
7   Cover with cling film and place in the fridge overnight.

The pâté can also be served with small triangles of toast with a salad garnish, tomato, lettuce, sliced cucumber and alfalfa sprouts. It keeps for four days in the fridge.

Pasta Salad

Use quantities to suit you: the amount given here will make enough for two children as well as for your own lunch. Don't worry about cooking too much as you can use it again for a day or two as long as it's refrigerated.

pasta, to taste, cooked according to the specifications on the packet
1 can of borlotti beans or red kidney beans

1 can of tuna (if there's any left over save the tuna for pizza on day 5)
1 onion, finely chopped
handful of parsley, chopped
lemon juice
olive oil

1   Drain and rinse the beans. In a mixing bowl, combine the beans, tuna, onion, pasta, a squeeze of lemon juice and a dash of olive oil.
2   Sprinkle with finely chopped parsley.

Melon Smiles

Cut a slice of melon (like an orange segment) and then, in that slice, make cuts through the melon flesh (but not through the skin) about every centimeter along. There you have a melon smile that is easier for your child to eat.

REFERENCES AND FURTHER READING

Breggin, Peter (2001) *Talking Back to Ritalin*. Perseus, ISBN 0-7382-0544-3. Read this book before your child is given Ritalin®.

Carter, Rita (2000) *Mapping the Mind*. Phoenix, ISBN 0-75381-019-0. A wonderful introduction to brain function.

Goddard, Sally (2002) *Reflexes, Learning and Behaviour: A window into the Child's Mind*. Fern Ridge Press, ISBN 0-9615332-8-5. A good book for those wishing to learn more about the primitive reflexes.

Haddon, Mark (2004) *The Curious Incident of the Dog in the Night-Time*. Vintage, ISBN 0-099-45025-9. A brilliant read to broaden your mind.

Hobart, Christine and Jill Frankel (2004) *A Practical Guide to Child Observation and Assessment*. Nelson Thornes, ISBN 0-7487-8526-4. A good starting point for those wishing to learn more about child development.

Holford, Patrick (2004) *Optimum Nutrition for the Mind*. Basic Health Publications, ISBN 1-59120-105-5. A good starting point if you want to learn more about improving your diet.

Jackson, Luke (2002) *Freaks, Geeks & Asperger Syndrome: A User Guide to Adolescence.* Jessica Kingsley Publishers, ISBN 1-84310-098-3. Asperger's as seen from the inside.

Lawrence, Felicity (2004) *Not on the Label.* Penguin Books, ISBN 0-141-01566-7. Find out what really goes into the food on your plate.

Meggitt, Carolyn and Gerald Sunderland (2000) *Child Development: Birth to 8 Years.* Heinemann, ISBN 0-435-42056-9. A pictorial reference guide.

Sheridan, Mary (1997) *From Birth to Five Years.* Routledge, ISBN 0-415-16458-3. A very basic guide to the early years.

Stordy, Jacqueline and Malcolm Nicholl (2002) *The LCP Solution.* Macmillan, ISBN 0-333-90622-5. Everything you need to know about long-chain polyunsaturated fatty acids.

INDEX